Mediterr___ ___an

Diet All-Time

Favorites

– Quick & Inspired Mediterranean

Diet Recipes for Beginners –

[Pamela Hartley]

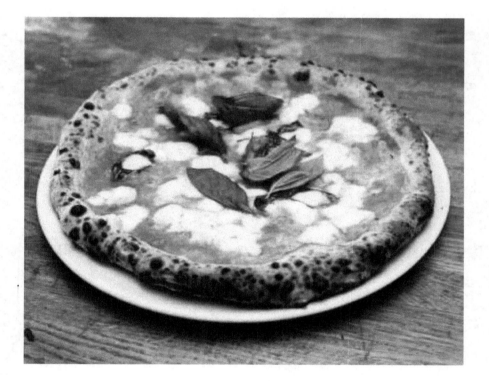

Table Of Content

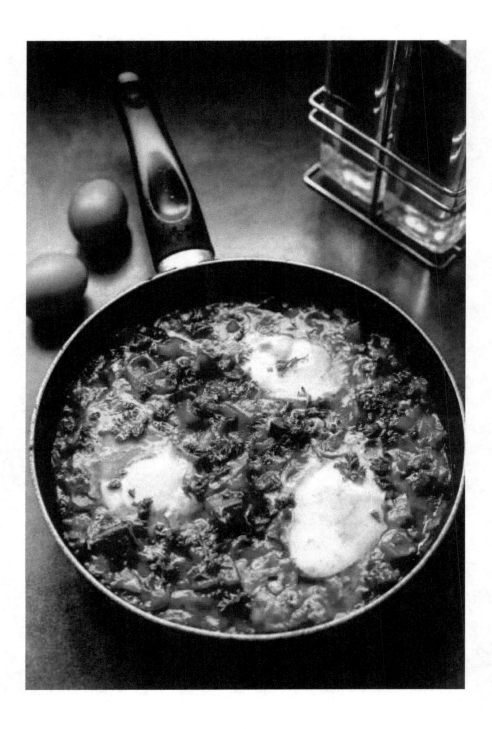

Additionally, the information in the following pages is intended only for informational purposes and should thus be thought of as universal. As befitting its nature, it is presented without assurance regarding its prolonged validity or interim quality. Trademarks that are mentioned are done without written consent and can in no way be considered an endorsement from the trademark holder.

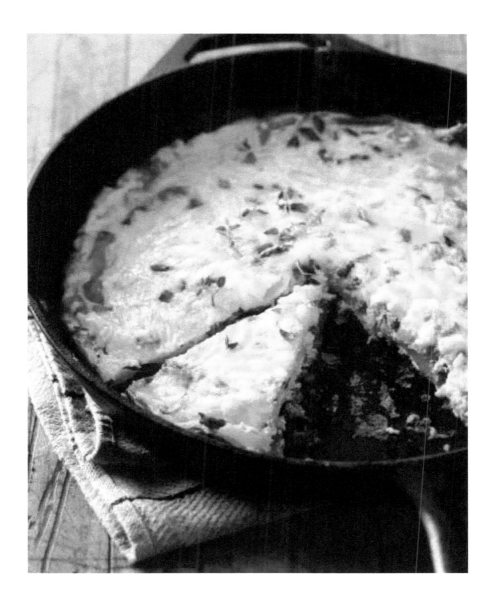

CHAPTER 1: **BREAKFAST**

Zucchini with Egg

Prep:

5 mins

Cook:

15 mins

Total:

20 mins

Servings:

2

Yield:

2 servings

Ingredients

1 ½ tablespoons olive oil
2 large eggs
salt and ground black pepper to taste
1 teaspoon water
2 large zucchini, cut into large chunks

Directions

1

Heat oil in a skillet over medium-high heat; saute zucchini until tender, about 12 minutes. Season zucchini with salt and black pepper.

2

Beat eggs with a fork in a bowl; add water and beat until evenly combined. Pour eggs over zucchini; cook and stir until eggs are scrambled and no longer runny, about 6 minutes. Season zucchini and eggs with salt and black pepper.

Nutrition
Per Serving:

213 calories; protein 10.2g; carbohydrates 11.2g; fat 15.7g; cholesterol 186mg; sodium 180mg.

Salad with Roquefort Cheese

Prep:

10 mins

Total:

10 mins

Servings:

8

Yield:

1 cheese ball

Ingredients

1 (8 ounce) package cream cheese, softened

2 tablespoons finely chopped celery

3 ounces crumbled blue cheese

3 drops hot pepper sauce (e.g. Tabasco™), or to taste

¾ cup finely chopped pecans

1 pinch cayenne pepper

2 tablespoons finely chopped onion

Directions

1

In a medium bowl, mix together the cream cheese and blue cheese. Blend in the celery, onion, hot pepper sauce, and cayenne pepper. Chill overnight, or until firm.

2

Roll the chilled cheese mixture into a ball, and coat with pecans. Wrap in waxed paper, and refrigerate until serving.

Nutrition

Per Serving: 207 calories; protein 5.4g; carbohydrates 2.7g; fat 20.1g; cholesterol 38.8mg; sodium 235mg

Lamb & Vegetable Bake

Prep:

30 mins

Cook:

1 hr

Total:

1 hr 30 mins

Servings:

6

Yield:

6 packages

Ingredients

aluminum foil
3 tablespoons minced garlic
salt and freshly ground black pepper to taste
6 (8 ounce) lamb shoulder chops
3 small zucchini, halved
6 small carrots, halved
2 sprigs chopped fresh rosemary
3 onions, sliced
6 tablespoons butter
8 ounces mushrooms, halved
1 (8 ounce) package feta cheese, cut into 6 squares
6 teaspoons freshly squeezed lemon juice

Directions

1

Preheat the oven to 375 degrees F.

2

Place 1 piece of heavy duty aluminum foil vertically on a work surface and 1 large piece aluminum foil horizontally on top, large enough to cover 1 lamb chop and vegetables..

3

Place 1 lamb chop in the middle of the aluminum foil and rub with 1/2 tablespoon garlic, salt, pepper, and rosemary. Repeat with remaining chops.

4

Stack zucchini, carrots, mushrooms, and onion on top of each lamb chop. Place 1 tablespoon of butter on top and drizzle with 1 teaspoon of lemon juice. Top each with 1 square of feta cheese. Tightly seal each package by wrapping the first piece of foil around the meat and vegetables, followed by the second.

5

Bake in the preheated oven until lamb is cooked but still pink in the center. An instant-read thermometer inserted into the center of a chop should read at least 140 degrees F. Serve each person their own individual parcel.

Nutrition
Per Serving:

715 calories; protein 43.1g; carbohydrates 21.1g; fat 51.1g; cholesterol 198.9mg; sodium 680.7mg

Sausage Pan

Prep:

25 mins

Cook:

25 mins

Total:

50 mins

Servings:

3

Yield:

3 servings

Ingredients

1 fresh mango, peeled and chopped
1 lime, juiced
1 tablespoon chopped red onion
½ fresh peach, peeled and chopped
2 cups water
1 cup white rice
½ cup orange juice
1 lime, juiced
1 tablespoon chopped fresh cilantro
3 Italian turkey sausage links
1 tablespoon chopped fresh cilantro
2 pinches garlic salt, or to taste
cooking spray

Directions

1

Place mango and peach in a small bowl. Squeeze juice of 1 lime over mango mixture; add onion and 1 tablespoon cilantro. Stir well.

2

Bring water to a boil in a saucepan over high heat. Add rice, juice of 1 lime, and 1 tablespoon cilantro; stir well. Reduce heat to medium-low, cover, and simmer until the rice is tender and the liquid has been absorbed, 16 to 20 minutes. Set rice aside and keep warm.

3

Spray a large nonstick skillet with cooking spray and place over medium heat. Cook and stir sausages in hot skillet until browned, 6 to 10 minutes. Remove sausages from pan; cut into bite-sized pieces.

4

Pour orange juice in skillet used for sausage; bring to a simmer. Return chopped sausage to skillet; cover and simmer in the orange juice until juice has reduced to a syrup and sausage is cooked through, about 5 minutes. Add mango salsa to sausage; stir to combine, about 40 seconds. Sprinkle with garlic salt; serve over rice.

Nutrition
Per Serving:

290 calories; protein 5.1g; carbohydrates 65.7g; fat 0.7g; sodium 231.1mg.

Peperoni Roasted in Oil

Prep:

10 mins

Cook:

20 mins

Total:

30 mins

Servings:

6

Yield:

6 servings

Ingredients

1 red bell pepper

5 leaves fresh basil leaves, finely sliced

1 orange bell pepper

¾ cup extra-virgin olive oil

1 yellow bell pepper

1 clove garlic, minced

½ teaspoon salt

¼ teaspoon ground black pepper

½ teaspoon dried oregano

Directions

1

Preheat an outdoor grill for high heat and lightly oil the grate. Reduce grill heat to medium.

2

Grill whole peppers until charred on all sides, turning about every 5 minutes. Place charred peppers in a plastic food storage bag and tie shut. Allow peppers to cool in bag.

3

Combine olive oil, garlic, basil, oregano, salt, and pepper in a 1-pint glass jar (or larger, depending on size of peppers).

4

Remove cooled peppers from bag and scrape off charred skins. Cut peppers in half and remove seeds and stems. Slice peppers into long strips and place in oil mixture. Mix well, assuring peppers are covered in oil. Serve, storing leftover peppers in refrigerator for up to 5 days.

Nutrition
Per Serving:

270 calories; protein 0.7g; carbohydrates 4g; fat 28.2g; sodium 195.5mg.

Menemen

Prep:

10 mins

Cook:

15 mins

Total:

25 mins

Servings:

2

Yield:

2 servings

Ingredients

1 tablespoon extra-virgin olive oil

2 tablespoons diced red bell pepper

1 tablespoon thinly sliced basil leaves

2 tablespoons diced Aleppo chiles, or to taste

½ teaspoon red pepper flakes

¼ cup chopped onion

1 teaspoon minced garlic

1 tablespoon crumbled feta cheese

salt and ground black pepper to taste

3 large eggs, beaten

¼ cup chopped tomato

Directions

1

Heat olive oil in a skillet over medium heat. Add onion, bell pepper, chiles, and red pepper flakes. Cook and stir until onions are soft and translucent, 5 to 7 minutes. Add garlic and cook until fragrant, about 1 minute. Add tomatoes, with their juices, and season with salt and pepper. Cook until tomatoes are softened, 5 to 6 minutes.

2

Add eggs to the skillet, tilting the skillet until eggs cover skillet completely. Do not mix. Cook until eggs are set, 4 to 5 minutes.

3

Top with basil and feta cheese.

Nutrition
Per Serving:

220 calories; protein 11.9g; carbohydrates 8.9g; fat 16.3g; cholesterol 283.2mg; sodium 162.9mg.

Avocado Toast

Prep:

10 mins

Cook:

4 mins

Total:

14 mins

Servings:

1

Yield:

1 serving

Ingredients

1 slice whole wheat bread

½ avocado

1 dash hot sauce (such as Cholula®)

½ teaspoon lime juice

¼ cup canned fat-free refried beans

1 pinch garlic powder

1 dash chili powder

1 dash salt

1 dash ground cumin

1 teaspoon pico de gallo

1 teaspoon crumbled queso fresco

1 egg

Directions

1

Toast whole wheat bread until golden brown. Spread refried beans on top.

2

Mash avocado in a small bowl; stir in lime juice, garlic powder, salt, chili powder, and cumin. Spread avocado over refried beans.

3

Heat a small nonstick skillet over medium heat. Crack egg into the skillet; cook until white is set, about 3 minutes. Cover skillet and cook until yolk is set, about 2 minutes more. Place egg over mashed avocado. Garnish with pico de gallo, queso fresco, and hot sauce.

Nutrition
Per Serving:

212 calories; protein 14.1g; carbohydrates 23.5g; fat 6.8g; cholesterol 187.7mg; sodium 952.9mg.

Berry Oat Muffins

Prep:

15 mins

Cook:

20 mins

Additional:

10 mins

Total:

45 mins

Servings:

12

Yield:

12 muffins

Ingredients

¾ cup rolled oats

1 ½ teaspoons baking powder

1 ½ cups all-purpose flour

¾ cup milk

½ cup white sugar

½ teaspoon baking soda

½ cup vegetable oil

1 egg, beaten

¼ teaspoon salt

1 tablespoon brown sugar

1 cup frozen saskatoon berries

Directions

1

Preheat oven to 350 degrees F. Grease a 12-cup muffin pan.

2

Stir oats and milk together in a small bowl; set aside.

3

Whisk flour, white sugar, baking powder, baking soda, and salt together in a large bowl. Whisk vegetable oil and egg together in a separate bowl; stir egg mixture into flour mixture just until batter is combined.

4

Fold oat mixture into batter; fold in saskatoon berries. Divide batter evenly into the prepared muffin cups; sprinkle muffins with brown sugar.

5

Bake in the preheated oven until a toothpick inserted into the center comes out clean, about 17 minutes. Cool in pans 10 minutes. Serve warm or cool completely on a wire rack.

Nutrition
Per Serving:

214 calories; protein 3.4g; carbohydrates 27.4g; fat 10.4g; cholesterol 16.7mg; sodium 175mg.

Cauliflower Fritters

Prep:

10 mins

Cook:

10 mins

Total:

20 mins

Servings:

6

Yield:

6 servings

Ingredients

3 extra large eggs

1 teaspoon baking powder

½ cup all-purpose flour

½ cup olive oil for frying

1 (.7 ounce) package dry Italian-style salad dressing mix

6 cups cauliflower florets

Directions

1

Process cauliflower in a food processor finely minced; transfer to a large bowl.

2

Stir flour, eggs, baking powder, and Italian dressing mix into cauliflower.

3

Heat enough olive oil to cover the bottom of a frying pan over medium heat.

4

Drop heaping tablespoons of cauliflower mixture into the hot oil; fry until golden brown, about 3 minutes per side.

Nutrition
Per Serving:

129 calories; protein 6.7g; carbohydrates 15.3g; fat 4.9g; cholesterol 107.9mg; sodium 682.2mg.

Chia Pineapple Smoothie

Prep:

10 mins

Total:

10 mins

Servings:

2

Yield:

2 smoothies

Ingredients

2 bananas

1 cup water

2 tablespoons almond butter

1 tablespoon chia seeds

1 cup frozen pineapple

Directions

1

Combine bananas, pineapple, almond butter, and chia seeds in a blender; add water. Blend until smooth.

Nutrition
Per Serving:

273 calories; protein 5g; carbohydrates 43.5g; fat 11.6g; sodium 78.6mg.

Shakshuka

Prep:

10 mins

Cook:

25 mins

Total:

35 mins

Servings:

2

Yield:

2 servings

Ingredients

2 teaspoons vegetable oil

1 onion, chopped

1 pinch salt

1 zucchini, chopped

2 cloves garlic, minced

4 dashes hot pepper sauce (such as Tabasco®)

4 eggs

1 (10 ounce) can crushed tomatoes

Directions

1

Heat the vegetable oil in a skillet over medium heat. Stir in the garlic and onion; cook and stir until the onion has softened and turned translucent, about 5 minutes. Stir in zucchini; cook and stir for 5-6 minutes. Mix in the crushed tomatoes and hot pepper sauce. Cover and simmer for 10-12 minutes.

2

Make 4 wells in the tomato mixture, and crack the eggs into each well. Do not stir. Cover and cook until eggs are desired consistency, about 3 minutes for soft yolks. Carefully remove the eggs from the skillet and serve with the tomato sauce.

Nutrition
Per Serving:

249 calories; protein 15.7g; carbohydrates 15.8g; fat 14.9g; cholesterol 372mg; sodium 442.9mg.

Goat Cheese Frittata Cups

Prep:

15 mins

Cook:

10 mins

Total:

25 mins

Servings:

30

Yield:

30 cups

Ingredients

2 eggs, beaten

¼ cup finely grated Parmigiano-Reggiano cheese

salt and ground black pepper to taste

2 (1.9 ounce) packages frozen miniature phyllo cups (such as Athen's®)

5 ounces goat cheese

1 (10 ounce) box frozen chopped spinach, thawed and drained

Directions

1

Preheat the oven to 350 degrees F.

2

Combine goat cheese, eggs, and Parmigiano-Reggiano cheese in a medium bowl with a spoon or fork. Add spinach and season with salt and pepper.

3

Space phyllo cups evenly on an ungreased cookie sheet. Spoon 1 heaping teaspoonful of the cheese mixture into each cup, pressing a bit to fit it in; mixture will not expand during baking.

4

Bake in the preheated oven until filling is hot and phyllo cups are lightly browned, 10 to 12 minutes. Serve warm.

Nutrition
Per Serving:

47 calories; protein 2.4g; carbohydrates 2.8g; fat 2.8g; cholesterol 15.2mg; sodium 59.8mg.

Spinach and Artichoke Frittata

Prep:

15 mins

Cook:

45 mins

Total:

1 hr

Servings:

12

Yield:

12 servings

Ingredients

1 (12 ounce) jar marinated artichoke hearts, drained and chopped (reserve marinade)
salt and ground black pepper to taste
9 eggs, beaten
1 pound sharp Cheddar cheese, grated
1 bunch green onions, chopped
14 saltine crackers, crumbled
2 cloves garlic, minced (Optional)
1 dash hot pepper sauce (such as Tabasco®)
½ cup chopped fresh parsley

Directions

1

Preheat oven to 325 degrees F.

2

Heat 3 tablespoons of the reserved marinade from the artichoke hearts in a large skillet. Cook and stir green onions in hot marinade until wilted, 2 to 4 minutes.

3

Stir cooked green onions, eggs, Cheddar cheese, saltine crackers, parsley, garlic, hot pepper sauce, salt, and black pepper together in a bowl; pour into a 9x13-inch baking dish.

4

Bake in the preheated oven until center is puffy and no longer moist, about 40 minutes; cool slightly before cutting into squares.

Nutrition

Per Serving:

265 calories; protein 15.4g; carbohydrates 8.7g; fat 19.2g; cholesterol 143.6mg; sodium 458.5mg.

Caprese Toast

Prep:

15 mins

Cook:

5 mins

Total:

20 mins

Servings:

14

Yield:

14 appetizers

Ingredients

14 slices sourdough bread
3 large tomatoes, sliced 1/4-inch thick
1 pound fresh mozzarella cheese, sliced 1/4-inch thick
⅓ cup fresh basil leaves
2 cloves garlic, peeled
salt and ground black pepper to taste
3 tablespoons extra-virgin olive oil

Directions

1

Toast bread slices and rub one side of each slice with garlic.
Place a slice of mozzarella cheese, 1 to 2 basil leaves, and a
slice of tomato on each piece of toast. Drizzle with olive oil
and season with salt and black pepper.

Nutrition
Per Serving:

204 calories; protein 10.5g; carbohydrates 16.5g; fat 10.7g; cholesterol 25.6mg; sodium 367.9mg.

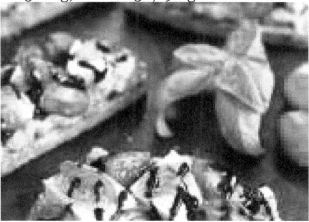

Homemade Muesli

Prep:

10 mins

Total:

10 mins

Servings:

8

Yield:

7 1/2 cups

Ingredients

½ cup coarsely chopped almonds
1 cup crispy rice cereal
½ cup dried cherries
½ cup golden raisins
½ cup raw sunflower seed kernels
4 cups whole oats
½ cup coarsely chopped pecans

Directions

1

Mix oats, rice cereal, pecans, almonds, sunflower seed kernels, dried cherries, and golden raisins together in a large bowl.

Nutrition

Per Serving:

361 calories; protein 10.2g; carbohydrates 49.1g; fat 15.3g; sodium 32.5mg.

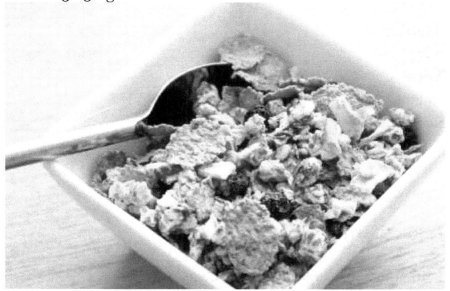

Gigantes

Prep:

10 mins

Cook:

1 hr 50 mins

Additional:

8 hrs

Total:

10 hrs

Servings:

8

Yield:

8 servings

Ingredients

1 (16 ounce) package dried lima beans
1 teaspoon chopped fresh dill
1 cup olive oil
3 cloves garlic, chopped
2 (16 ounce) cans chopped tomatoes with juice
sea salt to taste

Directions

1

Place the lima beans in a large saucepan. Pour enough water to fill to 2 inches above top of the beans. Allow to soak overnight.

2

Preheat oven to 375 degrees F.

3

Place the saucepan over medium heat; bring to a boil; reduce heat to medium-low and simmer 20 minutes; drain. Pour the beans into a 9 x 13 baking dish. Add the tomatoes, olive oil, garlic, salt, and dill; stir.

4

Bake in preheated oven for 1 1/2 to 2 hours, stirring occasionally and adding water if the mixture appears dry.

Nutrition
Per Serving:

449 calories; protein 13g; carbohydrates 40.4g; fat 27.5g; sodium 171mg.

Tuna Salad

Prep:

15 mins

Total:

15 mins

Servings:

4

Yield:

4 servings

Ingredients

2 (5 ounce) cans chunk light tuna in water, drained

2 tablespoons freshly squeezed lemon juice

¼ cup chopped fresh parsley

3 tablespoons olive oil

½ teaspoon lemon zest

¼ teaspoon ground black pepper

¼ teaspoon salt

¼ cup finely chopped red onion

Directions

1

Combine tuna, onion, and parsley in a medium bowl.

2

Whisk oil, lemon juice, lemon zest, salt, and pepper to make the dressing. Toss with the tuna mixture.

Nutrition
Per Serving:

169 calories; protein 16.3g; carbohydrates 1.6g; fat 10.7g; cholesterol 18.9mg; sodium 179.6mg.

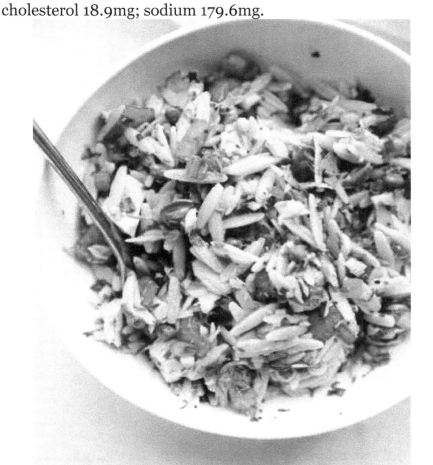

Yogurt Soup

Prep:

10 mins

Cook:

25 mins

Total:

35 mins

Servings:

4

Yield:

4 servings

Ingredients

4 cups whole milk
2 egg yolks
5 tablespoons all-purpose flour
2 cups water
3 cups plain yogurt
4 teaspoons chicken bouillon granules
1 teaspoon salt
2 tablespoons lemon juice
½ teaspoon ground black pepper

Directions

1

Beat milk, yogurt, egg yolks, and all-purpose flour in a large bowl with an electric mixer.

2

Meanwhile, bring water and chicken bouillon to a boil in a large soup pot. Reduce heat to medium-low and add yogurt mixture, lemon juice, salt, and pepper, stirring occasionally until mixture thickens, about 20 minutes.

Nutrition
Per Serving:

332 calories; protein 20.2g; carbohydrates 32.9g; fat 13.4g; cholesterol 138.1mg; sodium 1187.2mg.

Yogurt and Granola

Prep:

5 mins

Total:

5 mins

Servings:

1

Yield:

1 serving

Ingredients

¼ cup granola
1 tablespoon light agave syrup
1 (6 ounce) container fat-free plain yogurt
1 pinch ground cinnamon, or to taste
1 tablespoon flaxseed meal

Directions

1

Stir yogurt, granola, agave syrup, flaxseed meal, and cinnamon together in a bowl.

Nutrition
Per Serving:

344 calories; protein 15.6g; carbohydrates 48.1g; fat 10.6g; cholesterol 3.4mg; sodium 140.7mg.

Barley Porridge with Apple

Prep:

15 mins

Cook:

1 hr

Additional:

2 hrs

Total:

3 hrs 15 mins

Servings:

4

Yield:

4 servings

Ingredients

½ cup hulled barley

2 Golden Delicious apples - peeled, cored, and diced

2 cups water

1 cup water

2 teaspoons brown sugar

1 teaspoon butter

1 teaspoon lemon juice

1 teaspoon ground cinnamon

¼ teaspoon salt

½ cup chopped walnuts

¼ teaspoon ground nutmeg

Directions

1

Place barley in a bowl and add 1 cup water; soak for 2 hours or overnight. Drain.

2

Combine drained barley, apples, 2 cups water, brown sugar, cinnamon, butter, lemon juice, nutmeg, and salt in a saucepan; bring to a boil. Reduce heat to medium-low and simmer until barley and apples are softened and water is absorbed, adding more water if needed, about 60 minutes. Remove saucepan from heat and stir walnuts into barley.

Nutrition
Per Serving:

230 calories; protein 5.4g; carbohydrates 30.4g; fat 11.4g; cholesterol 2.7mg; sodium 163.1mg.

Blueberry Muffins

Prep:

10 mins

Cook:

35 mins

Total:

45 mins

Servings:

12

Yield:

1 dozen muffins

Ingredients

1 cooking spray

2 cups all-purpose flour

1 cup lightly packed brown sugar

2 cups fresh blueberries

½ cup soy milk

1 tablespoon baking powder

¼ cup soy margarine

1 teaspoon vanilla extract

½ teaspoon salt

½ cup unsweetened applesauce

Directions

1

Preheat the oven to 350 degrees F. Line 12 cups of a mini muffin tin with paper liners or spray with cooking spray.

2

Mix blueberries, flour, sugar, applesauce, soy milk, soy margarine, baking powder, vanilla extract, and salt together in a bowl. Spoon batter into muffin cups, filling them 3/4-full.

3

Bake in the preheated oven until tops are firm, about 35-40 minutes. Cool slightly on a rack.

Nutrition
Per Serving:

205 calories; protein 2.7g; carbohydrates 39.6g; fat 4.2g; sodium 274mg

Strawberry Muffins

Prep:

15 mins

Cook:

20 mins

Total:

35 mins

Servings:

12

Yield:

12 muffins

Ingredients

¾ cup white sugar

1 egg

1 ½ cups chopped strawberries

2 cups all-purpose flour

½ cup butter, softened

½ teaspoon salt

½ cup milk

2 teaspoons baking powder

½ teaspoon vanilla extract

½ teaspoon ground cinnamon

3 teaspoons white sugar

Directions

1

Preheat the oven to 400 degrees F. Grease a 12-cup muffin tin or line with paper liners.

2

Beat 3/4 cup sugar and butter together in a mixing bowl using an electric mixer until creamy. Add egg and mix well.

3

Sift flour, baking powder, and salt together in a small bowl. Add flour mixture and milk alternately to butter mixture until combined. Stir in vanilla extract. Gently stir in strawberries.

4

Spoon batter into the prepared muffin cups. Combine 3 teaspoons sugar and cinnamon in a small bowl and sprinkle over tops of muffins.

5

Bake in the preheated oven until a toothpick inserted into the center of a muffin comes out clean, 22 to 25 minutes.

Nutrition
Per Serving:

214 calories; protein 3.2g; carbohydrates 31.6g; fat 8.5g; cholesterol 36.6mg; sodium 243.3mg.

Flounder Mediterranean

Prep:

15 mins

Cook:

30 mins

Total:

45 mins

Servings:

4

Yield:

4 servings

Ingredients

5 roma (plum) tomatoes

2 tablespoons extra virgin olive oil

6 leaves fresh basil, torn

2 cloves garlic, chopped

1 pinch Italian seasoning

24 kalamata olives, pitted and chopped

½ Spanish onion, chopped

¼ cup white wine

¼ cup capers

6 leaves fresh basil, chopped

3 tablespoons freshly grated Parmesan cheese

1 teaspoon fresh lemon juice

1 pound flounder fillets

Directions

1

Preheat oven to 425 degrees F.

2

Bring a saucepan of water to a boil. Plunge tomatoes into the boiling water and immediately remove to a medium bowl of ice water; drain. Remove and discard skins from tomatoes. Chop tomatoes and set aside.

3

Heat olive oil in a skillet over medium heat; saute onion until tender, about 5 minutes. Stir in tomatoes, garlic and Italian seasoning; cook until tomatoes are tender, 6 to 7 minutes. Mix in olives, wine, capers, lemon juice, and 1/2 the basil. Reduce heat, blend in Parmesan cheese, and cook until the mixture is reduced to a thick sauce, about 15-17 minutes.

4

Place flounder in a shallow baking dish. Pour sauce over the fillets and top with remaining basil leaves.

5

Bake 12 minutes in the preheated oven, until fish is easily flaked with a fork.

Nutrition
Per Serving:

282 calories; protein 24.4g; carbohydrates 8.2g; fat 15.4g; cholesterol 63.5mg; sodium 777.5mg.

Grilled Honey-Nectarine Ricotta Toast

Prep:

10 mins

Cook:

10 mins

Additional:

5 mins

Total:

25 mins

Servings:

2

Yield:

2 servings

Ingredients

1 teaspoon olive oil

1 tablespoon crushed sliced almonds

2 thick slices crusty bread

2 teaspoons honey

2 tablespoons olive oil

1 large nectarine, pitted and cut into 8 wedges

¼ cup whole-milk ricotta cheese

2 leaves fresh mint, minced

Directions

1

Preheat an outdoor grill for medium-high heat and lightly oil grate.

2

Drizzle 1 teaspoon olive oil onto a small plate. Place nectarine wedges on the plate and cover all sides with oil. Brush both sides of bread with 2 tablespoons olive oil.

3

Place nectarines onto the hot grate and grill 1 to 2 minutes per side; remove to a plate. When nectarine wedges have cooled slightly, cut each wedge in 1/2 lengthwise so you now have 16 pieces.

4

Place bread slices onto the hot grate and cook until grill marks appear and bread is toasted, about 1 minute per side; remove to a plate.

5

Spread ricotta cheese onto each slice of toast. Arrange 8 nectarine slices onto each toast and top with almonds. Sprinkle with mint and drizzle with honey. Cut each toast in half and serve.

Nutrition

Per Serving:

336 calories; protein 7.3g; carbohydrates 31.7g; fat 20.9g; cholesterol 8.8mg; sodium 199.8mg.

Banana Corn Fritters

Prep:

10 mins

Cook:

10 mins

Total:

20 mins

Servings:

4

Yield:

8 to 10 fritters

Ingredients

⅓ cup dry bread crumbs

2 bananas, cut into bite-size pieces

2 tablespoons dry shredded coconut

¼ teaspoon ground cinnamon

1 egg white

1 teaspoon white sugar

Directions

1

Preheat oven to 350 degrees F. Line a baking sheet with parchment paper.

2

Combine bread crumbs, coconut, sugar, and cinnamon together in a bowl. Beat egg white in a small bowl until frothy. Dip each banana piece in egg white and press into bread crumb mixture. Place the breaded bananas on prepared baking sheet; do not stack.

3

Bake in preheated oven until golden brown, about 10 minutes.

Nutrition
Per Serving:

112 calories; protein 3g; carbohydrates 20.8g; fat 2.6g; sodium 81.4mg

Peach Smoothie

Prep:

5 mins

Total:

5 mins

Servings:

1

Yield:

1 smoothie

Ingredients

1 large peach, sliced and frozen

½ cup soy milk

½ cup orange juice

1 banana, cut into pieces and frozen

Directions

1

Blend peach, banana, orange juice, soy milk, and flax seed in a blender until smooth.

Nutrition

Per Serving:

297 calories; protein 7.4g; carbohydrates 57.5g; fat 5.7g; sodium 71.7mg.

Tzatziki

Prep:

40 mins

Additional:

1 hr

Total:

1 hr 40 mins

Servings:

10

Yield:

10 servings

Ingredients

¼ cup minced garlic

2 tablespoons lemon juice

1 ½ tablespoons red pepper flakes

4 ripe avocados, peeled and pitted

⅓ cup sour cream

1 cup diced English cucumber

⅓ cup plain yogurt

¼ cup chopped fresh dill

3 tablespoons chopped fresh cilantro

¼ cup chopped fresh mint

salt and ground black pepper to taste

Directions

1

Combine avocados, garlic, and lemon juice in a bowl; mash into a paste using a fork or spoon. Mix in yogurt and sour cream. Stir in cucumber, mint, dill, cilantro, red pepper flakes. Season with salt and pepper. Cover and refrigerate for at least 1 hour before serving.

Nutrition
Per Serving:

34 calories; protein 1.2g; carbohydrates 3.5g; fat 2g; cholesterol 3.9mg; sodium 27.2mg.

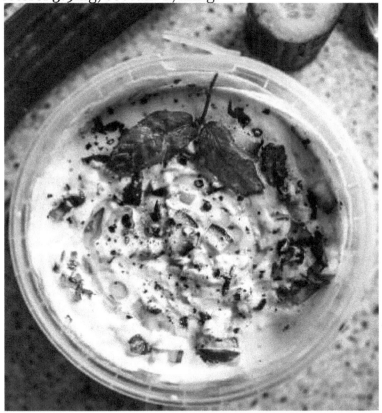

Iced Coffee

Prep:

10 mins

Cook:

20 mins

Additional:

4 hrs

Total:

4 hrs 30 mins

Servings:

8

Yield:

8 servings

Ingredients

1 ½ quarts brewed coffee, room temperature
1 cup milk
2 tablespoons creme de cacao
⅓ cup white sugar
1 teaspoon vanilla extract
1 cup half-and-half cream

Directions

1

In a pitcher, combine cooled coffee, milk and half-and-half.
Stir in sugar, vanilla and creme de cacao. Chill in refrigerator
until ready to serve.

Nutrition

Per Serving:

106 calories; protein 2.1g; carbohydrates 13.1g; fat 4.1g; cholesterol 13.6mg; sodium 28.8mg.

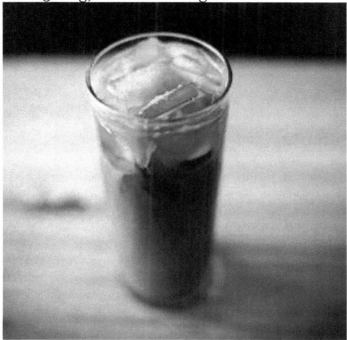

Muesli

Prep:

10 mins

Total:

10 mins

Servings:

16

Yield:

8 cups

Ingredients

½ cup toasted wheat germ

½ cup chopped walnuts

½ cup wheat bran

¼ cup packed brown sugar

¼ cup raw sunflower seeds

½ cup oat bran

4 ½ cups rolled oats

1 cup raisins

Directions

1

In a large mixing bowl combine oats, wheat germ, wheat bran, oat bran, dried fruit, nuts, sugar, and seeds. Mix well. Store muesli in an airtight container. It keeps for 2 months at room temperature.

Nutrition
Per Serving:

188 calories; protein 6.1g; carbohydrates 31.8g; fat 5.7g; sodium 3.9mg.

Cheesy Rice Bites

Prep:

10 mins

Cook:

20 mins

Total:

30 mins

Servings:

8

Yield:

24 bites

Ingredients

1 (8.8 ounce) pouch UNCLE BEN'S® Ready Rice® Original
Long Grain

1 ½ cups shredded Cheddar-Monterey Jack cheese blend

1 ½ cups prepared pulled pork in barbeque sauce

2 eggs

1 (15 ounce) can black beans, rinsed and drained

Directions

1

Preheat oven to 400 degrees F. Spray mini muffin tin cups
with cooking spray.

2

Prepare rice according to package directions. Allow to cool
slightly. Combine rice, black beans, barbeque pulled pork,
cheese, and eggs in a bowl; mix well.

3

Drop mixture by heaping tablespoons into prepared mini muffin tins, filling each cup to the top.

4

Bake in preheated oven until hot, about 20-22 minutes.

5

Allow bites to cool 6 to 10 minutes before popping them out of the muffin tin.

Nutrition

Per Serving:

298 calories; protein 18.8g; carbohydrates 25.5g; fat 13.4g; cholesterol 81.3mg; sodium 612.6mg.

Garlicky Mushrooms

Prep:

20 mins

Cook:

30 mins

Additional:

15 mins

Total:

1 hr 5 mins

Servings:

6

Yield:

6 toast cups

Ingredients

1 tablespoon butter

3 tablespoons freshly grated Parmesan cheese

12 ounces sliced mushrooms

1 teaspoon salt

½ teaspoon black pepper

2 cloves garlic, minced

2 tablespoons softened butter

3 eggs, beaten

2 tablespoons cream

6 firm white or wheat bread, crusts removed

Directions

1

Preheat oven to 350 degrees F.

2

Melt 1 tablespoon of butter in a large skillet over medium-high heat. Stir in garlic, and cook for 30 seconds until fragrant. Add mushrooms, and continue cooking until softened and lightly browned, 5 to 6 minutes. Season with salt and pepper, then set aside to cool.

3

Meanwhile, spread softened butter onto one side of each slice of bread. Press the buttered sides into a muffin tin; set aside.

4

Stir together eggs and cream, then stir in the cooled mushroom mixture. Divide this custard equally among the toast cups. Sprinkle the tops with grated Parmesan cheese.

5

Bake in preheated oven until egg mixture sets, and tops are golden brown, about 20 minutes.

Nutrition

Per Serving: 161 calories; protein 7g; carbohydrates 8.8g; fat 11.4g; cholesterol 117.3mg; sodium 588.4mg.

Parmesan Spinach Pie

Prep:

10 mins

Cook:

35 mins

Total:

45 mins

Servings:

6

Yield:

6 servings

Ingredients

¼ teaspoon Italian seasoning

6 skinless, boneless chicken breasts

⅓ cup grated Parmesan cheese

¼ cup chopped green onions

1 tablespoon all-purpose flour

1 tablespoon chopped pimento peppers

½ cup skim milk

1 tablespoon butter

½ (10 ounce) package frozen chopped spinach, thawed and drained

Directions

1

Preheat oven to 350 degrees F.

2

In a small bowl combine cheese and seasoning. Roll chicken pieces in cheese mixture to coat lightly. Set remaining cheese mixture aside. Arrange coated chicken pieces in an 8x8x2 inch baking dish.

3

In a small saucepan, saute green onion in butter/margarine until tender. Stir in flour, then add milk all at once. Simmer, stirring, until bubbly. Stir in drained spinach and pimiento and mix together. Spoon spinach mixture over chicken and sprinkle with remaining cheese mixture. Bake uncovered for 30 to 35 minutes or until tender and chicken juices run clear.

Nutrition
Per Serving:

187 calories; protein 30.8g; carbohydrates 3.6g; fat 4.8g; cholesterol 77.8mg; sodium 185.4mg.

Chia Seeds Jam

Prep:

10 mins

Cook:

15 mins

Additional:

10 mins

Total:

35 mins

Servings:

10

Yield:

10 servings

Ingredients

½ cup water
2 cups frozen raspberries
¼ cup chia seeds
½ cup frozen blackberries
2 frozen strawberries, or more to taste
⅓ cup honey
½ cup frozen blueberries

Directions

1

Soak chia seeds in water until mixture has a jelly-like texture, about 6 minutes.

2

Heat raspberries, blackberries, blueberries, strawberries, and honey in a saucepan over medium heat until berries are soft, about 15 minutes. Lightly crush berries with a fork or masher.

3

Stir chia seed mixture into berry mixture. Remove from heat and let cool for at least 10 minutes.

Nutrition
Per Serving:

70 calories; protein 1g; carbohydrates 15.3g; fat 1g; sodium 1.9mg.

CHAPTER 2: LUNCH

Asparagus Pasta

Prep:

5 mins

Cook:

25 mins

Total:

30 mins

Servings:

8

Yield:

8 servings

Ingredients

1 pound fresh asparagus, trimmed and cut into 2 inch pieces
1 lemon, juiced
1 clove garlic, minced
1 pint light cream
2 tablespoons butter
1 pound linguine pasta

Directions

1

Bring a pot of water to a boil. Boil asparagus for 3 to 4 minutes; drain.

2

In a large saucepan melt butter over medium heat. Saute garlic and asparagus for 3 to 4 minutes. Stir in the cream and simmer for 10 minutes.

3

Meanwhile, bring a large pot of water to a boil. Add linguine and cook for 8 to 10 minutes or until al dente; drain and transfer to a serving dish.

4

Stir lemon juice into asparagus mixture; pour mixture over pasta.

Nutrition
Per Serving:

247 calories; protein 8.3g; carbohydrates 44g; fat 4.7g; cholesterol 9.9mg; sodium 30.9mg.

Bulgarian Moussaka

Prep:

30 mins

Cook:

1 hr 30 mins

Total:

2 hrs

Servings:

12

Yield:

12 servings

Ingredients

¾ pound ground beef (85% lean)

¾ pound ground pork

1 large carrot, finely chopped

½ yellow onion, finely chopped

½ cup olive oil, divided

2 stalks celery, finely chopped

1 (14.5 ounce) can diced tomatoes

1 red bell pepper, finely chopped

¼ bunch fresh parsley, stems and leaves chopped separately

2 tablespoons paprika

1 tablespoon salt

2 bay leaves

½ teaspoon cayenne pepper

1 teaspoon black pepper

6 russet potatoes, peeled and cut into 1/2-inch dice

Topping:

2 eggs

2 cups plain yogurt

1 teaspoon baking soda

¼ cup all-purpose flour

Directions

1

Heat a large skillet over medium heat. Add ground beef and ground pork and cook until brown and crumbly, 5 to 10 minutes. Drain and discard fat. Add 1/4 cup olive oil, carrot, onion, celery, parsley stems, and tomatoes. Mix to combine. Stir in bell pepper and season with paprika, salt, pepper, bay leaves, and cayenne pepper. Cook until vegetables start to soften, about 10 minutes.

2

Meanwhile, preheat the oven to 400 degrees F.

3

Transfer meat mixture to a large baking pan.

4

Heat remaining 1/4 cup olive oil in a large skillet and cook potatoes until lightly browned, about 10 minutes. Transfer to the baking pan and mix well with the meat mixture.

5

Bake moussaka in the preheated oven for 45 minutes. Remove baking dish from the oven and mix in chopped parsley leaves.

6

Stir eggs, yogurt, flour, and baking soda together in a bowl until it turns into a spreadable mixture. Pour over the meat mixture in the baking dish.

7

Return baking dish to the oven and cook until the top is golden brown, about 15 more minutes.

Nutrition
Per Serving:

335 calories; protein 16.4g; carbohydrates 27.7g; fat 17.8g; cholesterol 72.4mg; sodium 829.4mg.

Tomato Salad

Prep:

10 mins

Additional:

5 mins

Total:

15 mins

Servings:

4

Yield:

4 servings

Ingredients

2 cups halved grape tomatoes

1 tablespoon sweetened rice vinegar

¼ teaspoon garlic powder

1 tablespoon olive oil

1 pinch salt to taste

¼ teaspoon dried oregano

Directions

1

Mix tomatoes, olive oil, rice vinegar, and garlic powder together in a bowl. Crumble oregano between fingers to release flavor and add to the tomatoes; stir to coat. Season with salt. Let flavors marinate before serving, 5 minutes or up to an hour.

Nutrition

Per Serving:

47 calories; protein 0.8g; carbohydrates 3.7g; fat 3.6g; sodium 4.6mg.

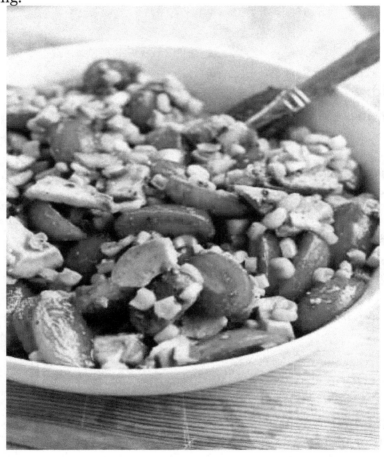

Parmesan Risotto with Truffle

Prep:

20 mins

Cook:

30 mins

Total:

50 mins

Servings:

4

Yield:

4 servings

Ingredients

1 quart chicken broth
1 tablespoon olive oil
½ onion, minced
1 tablespoon butter
½ cup white wine
2 tablespoons butter
2 tablespoons white truffle oil
⅓ cup grated Parmesan cheese
1 ¼ cups Arborio rice
1 teaspoon milk
2 tablespoons chopped fresh parsley
salt and ground black pepper to taste

Directions

1

Heat chicken broth in a stockpot over medium-low heat until warmed.

2

Heat 1 tablespoon butter and olive oil in a large, heavy-bottomed pan; cook and stir onion in the melted butter-oil mixture until translucent, about 2 minutes. Add rice to onion mixture and stir to coat; cook and stir rice mixture until fragrant, about 1 minute.

3

Pour wine into rice mixture; cook and stir until liquid is absorbed, about 5 minutes. Add 1 ladle of hot chicken broth to rice mixture, stirring constantly, until broth is absorbed. Continue adding 1 ladle of broth at a time until rice is tender but firm to the bite, 20 to 30 minutes.

4

Mix 2 tablespoons butter, truffle oil, Parmesan cheese, and milk into risotto until fully incorporated; season with salt, pepper, and parsley.

Nutrition
Per Serving:

498 calories; protein 8.6g; carbohydrates 60.5g; fat 21.4g; cholesterol 33.8mg; sodium 1126.5mg.

Beef Tartar

Prep:

15 mins

Total:

15 mins

Servings:

4

Yield:

4 servings

Ingredients

1 ½ tablespoons Worcestershire sauce

1 tablespoon Dijon mustard

2 dashes hot pepper sauce (such as Tabasco®), or more to taste

½ tablespoon capers, roughly chopped

10 ½ ounces beef filet, finely chopped by hand

¼ teaspoon curry powder, or to taste

2 teaspoons olive oil

2 tablespoons ketchup

1 pinch salt

1 pinch ground black pepper

2 tablespoons finely chopped onion

2 tablespoons finely chopped gherkin pickles

4 anchovy fillets

2 egg yolks

¼ cup beer

Directions

1

Put olive oil in a serving bowl. Add ketchup, Worcestershire sauce, Dijon mustard, hot pepper sauce, curry powder, curry powder, salt, and ground pepper. Mix thoroughly.

2

Crush anchovy fillets on a plate using 2 forks until they are finely separated. Add onion, gherkin, and capers; stir together before scraping into the bowl with the ketchup mixture. Add chopped beef; mix thoroughly. Stir in egg yolks and beer.

Nutrition
Per Serving:

298 calories; protein 16g; carbohydrates 6.8g; fat 22.2g; cholesterol 158.7mg; sodium 526.2mg.

Chicken Salad

Prep:

15 mins

Cook:

15 mins

Total:

30 mins

Servings:

2

Yield:

2 servings

Ingredients

2 skinless, boneless chicken breast halves

2 tablespoons chopped fresh cilantro

1 avocado, diced

4 scallions, chopped

¼ sweet onion, chopped

½ lime, juiced

1 stalk celery, chopped

salt and ground black pepper to taste

Directions

1

Preheat oven to 375 degrees F. Line a baking sheet with aluminum foil.

2

Place chicken breasts on prepared baking sheet.

3

Cook in the preheated oven until no longer pink in the middle and juices run clear, 15 to 20 minutes. An instant-read thermometer inserted into the center should read at least 165 degrees F. Shred chicken breasts.

4

Stir chicken, avocado, scallions, celery, onion, lime juice, cilantro, cayenne pepper, salt, and black pepper together in a bowl.

Nutrition
Per Serving:

338 calories; protein 32.1g; carbohydrates 13.6g; fat 18.2g; cholesterol 79.9mg; sodium 99.5mg

Cauliflower Salad with Tahini

Prep:

10 mins

Cook:

35 mins

Total:

45 mins

Servings:

4

Yield:

4 servings

Ingredients

Cauliflower:
2 tablespoons olive oil, divided
1 teaspoon salt
Tahini Sauce:
2 tablespoons plain yogurt
1 tablespoon tahini
1 head cauliflower, broken into florets
2 teaspoons za'atar
1 tablespoon lemon juice
1 tablespoon warm water
salt to taste
Garnish:
1 tablespoon sesame seeds

Directions

1

Preheat the oven to 400 degrees F. Grease a baking sheet lightly with 1 tablespoon olive oil.

2

Place cauliflower florets into a bowl and toss with remaining 1 tablespoon olive oil, za'atar, and salt. Arrange in a single layer on the prepared baking sheet.

3

Bake in the preheated oven until golden brown, 37 to 42 minutes, turning after 20 minutes.

4

Prepare the tahini sauce while the cauliflower is roasting. Mix yogurt, tahini, and lemon juice in a small bowl until well combined. Stir in warm water, 1 tablespoon at a time, until a drizzling consistency is achieved. Season with more salt or lemon juice if desired.

5

Place sesame seeds in a small skillet over medium heat. Toast, stirring often, until golden, about 3 minutes. Remove from the skillet.

6

Arrange cauliflower in an even layer in a shallow dish, drizzle with

Nutrition

Per Serving:

139 calories; protein 4.4g; carbohydrates 10.4g; fat 10.2g; cholesterol 0.5mg; sodium 674mg.

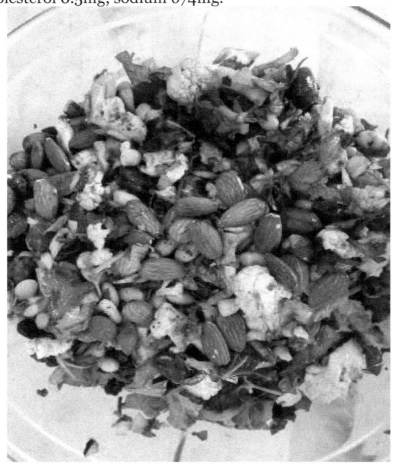

Cobb Salad

Prep:

20 mins

Cook:

30 mins

Total:

50 mins

Servings:

6

Yield:

6 servings

Ingredients

6 slices bacon

3 eggs

1 head iceberg lettuce, shredded

1 (8 ounce) bottle Ranch-style salad dressing

2 tomatoes, seeded and chopped

¾ cup blue cheese, crumbled

3 cups chopped, cooked chicken meat

3 green onions, chopped

1 avocado - peeled, pitted and diced

Directions

1

Place eggs in a saucepan and cover completely with cold water. Bring water to a boil. Cover, remove from heat, and let eggs stand in hot water for 10 to 12 minutes. Remove from hot water, cool, peel and chop.

2

Place bacon in a large, deep skillet. Cook over medium high heat until evenly brown. Drain, crumble and set aside.

3

Divide shredded lettuce among individual plates.

4

Evenly divide and arrange chicken, eggs, tomatoes, blue cheese, bacon, avocado and green onions in a row on top of the lettuce.

5

Drizzle with your favorite dressing and enjoy.

Nutrition
Per Serving:

525 calories; protein 31.7g; carbohydrates 10.2g; fat 39.9g; cholesterol 179.1mg; sodium 915.2mg

Red Onion Tilapia

Prep:

10 mins

Cook:

15 mins

Additional:

2 mins

Total:

27 mins

Servings:

1

Yield:

1 tilapia fillet

Ingredients

¼ large lemon

salt and ground black pepper to taste

1 tablespoon grated fresh Parmesan cheese

1 tablespoon extra-virgin olive oil

1 (6 ounce) tilapia fillet, patted dry

1 teaspoon butter, divided

1 teaspoon minced garlic

¼ large red onion, coarsely chopped

Directions

1

Squeeze lemon juice over tilapia; season lightly with salt and black pepper.

2

Heat olive oil in a nonstick skillet over medium heat. Melt 1/2 teaspoon butter in hot oil. Add chopped onion and minced garlic; cook and stir until onion begins to look translucent, about 5 minutes.

3

Reduce heat to medium-low. Push onion mixture to sides of the skillet. Melt remaining 1/2 teaspoon of butter in the skillet. Place tilapia in the center of the skillet and cover with onion mixture. Cover skillet and cook tilapia until it starts to turn golden, about 5 minutes. Push onion mixture to the sides again and flip tilapia. Cover and cook until second side is golden and flakes easily with a fork, about 5 minutes more.

4

Remove skillet from heat. Top tilapia with grated Parmesan cheese, cover, and let stand until cheese is melted, about 3 minutes.

Nutrition
Per Serving:

371 calories; protein 37.3g; carbohydrates 7.6g; fat 21.4g; cholesterol 76.7mg; sodium 337.8mg.

Beef Kofta

Prep:

20 mins

Cook:

10 mins

Total:

30 mins

Servings:

4

Yield:

4 servings

Ingredients

1 pound ground beef
1 onion, diced
2 tablespoons chopped fresh oregano
salt and pepper to taste
1 egg yolk
1 bamboo skewers, soaked in water for 20 minutes

Directions

1

In a medium bowl, mix together the ground beef, onion, egg yolk, oregano, salt and pepper.

2

Pick up medium sized handfuls and press them onto skewers. Roll on a lightly oiled clean surface until the mixture looks like a large ground beef hot dog with about 1 1/2 inches at each end of the skewer. Place your fingers in the middle of the skewer and separate the meat log into two sausages with about 1 inch of skewer sticking out at each end.

3

Prepare a grill for high heat, or if you only have a grill pan, like myself, heat it over medium-high heat.

4

Place the sausages on the grilling surface, and cook for about 10 minutes, turning once or twice for even cooking. Serve immediately.

Nutrition
Per Serving:

231 calories; protein 20.5g; carbohydrates 2.7g; fat 14.8g; cholesterol 122mg; sodium 70.3mg.

Chicken Alfredo Casserole

Prep:

15 mins

Cook:

45 mins

Total:

1 hr

Servings:

6

Yield:

6 servings

Ingredients

3 skinless, boneless chicken breast halves
1 cup shredded Cheddar cheese
1 (8 ounce) package penne pasta
½ (16 ounce) jar Alfredo sauce
1 ½ cups shredded mozzarella cheese, divided
¼ cup milk
1 tablespoon garlic powder
1 tablespoon onion powder

Directions

1

Preheat the oven to 350 degrees F.

2

Place chicken into a pot and cover with water. Bring to a boil over high heat; reduce heat and simmer until no longer pink in the centers and juices run clear, about 15 minutes.

3

At the same time, bring a large pot of lightly salted water to a boil. Add penne and cook, stirring occasionally, until tender yet firm to the bite, about 11 minutes. Drain. Drain cooked chicken and cut into bite-size pieces.

4

Place chicken, noodles, Alfredo sauce, 1/2 mozzarella cheese, milk, onion powder, and garlic powder in a large bowl and mix well. Pour into a 1 1/2-quart casserole dish. Layer remaining mozzarella cheese and Cheddar cheese on top.

5

Bake in the preheated oven until melted and bubbly, about 25 minutes.

Nutrition
Per Serving:

468 calories; protein 30.8g; carbohydrates 32.4g; fat 24.2g; cholesterol 86.2mg; sodium 693.4mg.

Chicken Korma

Prep:

20 mins

Cook:

7 hrs 15 mins

Total:

7 hrs 35 mins

Servings:

4

Yield:

4 servings

Ingredients

2 onions, quartered

5 tablespoons heavy cream

1 large green chile pepper, seeded

3 cloves garlic

1 tablespoon white sugar

1 ½ inch piece fresh ginger root, peeled

8 boneless, skinless chicken thighs

2 tablespoons butter

1 teaspoon cumin seeds, crushed

1 tablespoon sunflower seed oil

1 teaspoon fennel seeds, crushed

1 teaspoon paprika

1 teaspoon ground turmeric

¼ teaspoon ground cinnamon

4 cardamom pods, crushed

11 ounces chicken stock

1 pinch salt

2 tablespoons ground almonds

Directions

1

Combine onions, chile pepper, garlic, and ginger in a blender; blend until smooth. Cut each chicken thigh into 4 pieces.

2

Heat oil in a large skillet over high heat and brown chicken pieces in batches until evenly browned on all sides, about 5 minutes per batch. Transfer to a slow cooker.

3

Melt butter in the same skillet over medium heat and add onion mixture once butter has melted. Cook until flavors are well combined, about 3 minutes. Stir in cumin, fennel, cardamom, paprika, turmeric, and cinnamon and cook for 1 minute more. Mix in chicken stock, sugar, and salt; bring to a boil. Pour contents of skillet over chicken in the slow cooker. Cover.

4

Cook on Low until chicken is cooked through and flavors are well combined, about 7 hours. Stir in heavy cream and ground almonds.

Nutrition
Per Serving:

436 calories; protein 25.1g; carbohydrates 15g; fat 31.1g; cholesterol 118.5mg; sodium 384.2mg.

Chicken Souvlaki

20 mins
Cook:
10 mins
Additional:
2 hrs
Total:
2 hrs 30 mins
Servings:
4
Yield:
4 servings

Ingredients

1 tablespoon olive oil
1 lemon, juiced
2 cloves garlic, finely grated or minced
1 tablespoon Greek seasoning
1 pound boneless chicken breasts, quartered lengthwise
½ English cucumber, sliced
2 tablespoons olive oil
2 tablespoons fresh lemon juice
1 pinch salt
1 head romaine, trimmed, washed and torn into bite-sized pieces
½ cup thinly sliced red bell pepper
6 tablespoons tzatziki sauce
8 ounces cherry tomatoes, halved

Directions

1

Combine 1 tablespoon olive oil, Greek seasoning, lemon juice, and garlic in a glass bowl; mix well. Add chicken to marinade and turn to coat. Marinate in the refrigerator for at least 2 hours, but not longer than 4 hours.

2

Mix tzatziki, 2 tablespoons olive oil, 2 tablespoons lemon juice, and salt in a small bowl. Refrigerate salad dressing until needed.

3

Preheat an outdoor grill for high heat and lightly oil the grate.

4

Place chicken pieces on the grill and cook for 5 minutes, turn, and grill until no longer pink in the center and the juices run clear, about 5 more minutes. An instant-read thermometer inserted into the centers should read at least 165 degrees F.

5

Combine romaine lettuce, bell pepper, cucumber, and cherry tomatoes in a salad bowl. Drizzle with tzatziki dressing and toss to coat. Divide salad into 4 equal portions and top with cooked chicken.

Nutrition
Per Serving:

287 calories; protein 26.8g; carbohydrates 13.9g; fat 32.3g; cholesterol 64.6mg; sodium 483.6mg

Spicy Chicken Shawarma

Prep:

15 mins

Cook:

10 mins

Total:

25 mins

Servings:

4

Yield:

4 shawarmas

Ingredients

1 clove garlic, minced

4 dill pickle spears

2 large skinless, boneless chicken breast halves - cut into bite-size pieces

1 ½ teaspoons garam masala

4 pita bread rounds

½ cup mayonnaise

2 tablespoons unsalted butter

Directions

1

Stir together the garlic and mayonnaise in a small bowl; set aside. Heat the butter in a skillet over medium-high heat. Cook and stir the chicken in the hot butter until white on the outside. Sprinkle with garam masala, and continue cooking until lightly browned on the outside and no longer pink in the center, about 4 minutes.

2

Spread the pita rounds with the garlic mayonnaise. Divide the chicken among the pitas, and place a pickle spear into each. Fold and serve.

Nutrition
Per Serving:

516 calories; protein 31.2g; carbohydrates 29.7g; fat 29.8g; cholesterol 91.6mg; sodium 590.6mg.

Sausage Marsala

Prep:

20 mins

Cook:

20 mins

Total:

40 mins

Servings:

6

Yield:

6 servings

Ingredients

1 (16 ounce) package farfalle (bow tie) pasta

1 pound mild Italian sausage links

1 pinch black pepper

1 clove garlic, minced

½ large onion, sliced

⅓ cup water

1 medium green bell pepper, sliced

1 tablespoon Marsala wine

1 (14.5 ounce) can Italian-style diced tomatoes, undrained

1 medium red bell pepper, sliced

1 pinch dried oregano

Directions

1

Bring a large pot of lightly salted water to a boil. Cook pasta for 10 minutes, or until al dente; drain.

2

Place whole sausages and 1/3 cup water in a skillet over medium-high heat. Cover, and cook 6 to 7 minutes. Drain and thinly slice.

3

Return sausage to skillet. Stir in garlic, onions, peppers, and Marsala wine. Cook over medium-high heat, stirring frequently, until sausage is cooked through. Stir in diced tomatoes, black pepper, and oregano. Cook about 2 minutes more, then remove from heat. Serve over cooked pasta.

Nutrition
Per Serving:

510 calories; protein 21.9g; carbohydrates 66.1g; fat 16.1g; cholesterol 29.8mg; sodium 740.6mg.

Orzo Primavera

Prep:

15 mins

Cook:

30 mins

Total:

45 mins

Servings:

6

Yield:

6 servings

Ingredients

4 teaspoons kosher salt, divided

1 tablespoon olive oil

1 red bell pepper, chopped

½ cup grated Parmesan cheese

1 ⅓ cups uncooked orzo pasta

1 carrot, cut into thin slices

1 tablespoon minced garlic

1 medium zucchini, cut into bite-sized pieces

1 medium onion, chopped

½ cup chicken broth

½ cup tomato sauce

¼ teaspoon ground black pepper

2 tablespoons half-and-half

1 medium yellow squash, cut into bite-sized pieces

Directions

1

Bring a large pot of water to a rolling boil; add 2 teaspoons salt. Cook orzo in the boiling water, stirring occasionally until tender yet firm to the bite, 6 to 10 minutes. Drain.

2

Heat oil in a skillet over low heat. Add bell pepper and saute for 10 minutes. Increase heat to medium and add carrot, onion, and garlic. Saute until carrot begins to soften, about 3 minutes. Add zucchini and summer squash; cook for 1 minute more. Increase heat to high and add broth, tomato sauce, remaining salt, and pepper. Cook until sauce comes to a simmer, about 5 minutes. Reduce heat to low.

3

Add orzo to the sauce and mix well. Remove from heat. Stir in half-and-half, followed by Parmesan cheese. Serve hot or at room temperature.

Nutrition

Per Serving: 253 calories; protein 10.4g; carbohydrates 41.3g; fat 5.7g; cholesterol 8.2mg; sodium 1602.7mg.

Citrus-Herb Scallops

Prep:

30 mins

Cook:

15 mins

Total:

45 mins

Servings:

4

Yield:

4 servings

Ingredients

2 tablespoons olive oil

4 green onions, thinly sliced

4 large oranges, peeled and segmented

1 tablespoon chopped fresh cilantro

1 clove garlic, minced

1 red bell pepper, thinly sliced

1 pound scallops

½ tablespoon salt

½ teaspoon grated lime zest

2 tablespoons fresh lime juice

¼ teaspoon crushed red pepper flakes

Directions

1

In a large skillet, heat the oil over medium-high heat. Add the red bell pepper, green onions and garlic. Cook, stirring for 1 minute. Add the scallops, salt and red pepper flakes. Cook until the scallops are opaque and the red bell pepper is tender, about 4 to 6 minutes.

2

Stir in the lime zest and juice, scraping up any browned bits from the bottom of the skillet. Cook for 1 minute. Add the oranges and cilantro, cook until heated through, about 2 minutes.

Nutrition
Per Serving:

264 calories; protein 21.5g; carbohydrates 28.3g; fat 8g; cholesterol 37.5mg; sodium 1059.2mg.

Tomato Spaghetti

Prep:

15 mins

Cook:

1 hr 10 mins

Total:

1 hr 25 mins

Servings:

8

Yield:

1 quart sauce

Ingredients

¼ cup olive oil

1 onion, chopped

1 tablespoon white sugar

1 tablespoon dried basil

½ teaspoon garlic powder

4 pounds fresh tomatoes, peeled and chopped

1 teaspoon salt

1 tablespoon dried parsley

Directions

1

Heat olive oil in a large skillet over medium heat. Add onion and garlic powder; cook and stir until onion is translucent, about 5 minutes. Add tomatoes, sugar, basil, parsley, and salt. Bring to a boil. Reduce heat and simmer, stirring occasionally, until sauce thickens, 1 to 2 hours.

Nutrition
Per Serving:

120 calories; protein 2.5g; carbohydrates 13.5g; fat 7.3g; sodium 304.3mg.

.

Spice Burgers

Prep:

5 mins

Total:

5 mins

Servings:

20

Yield:

20 servings

Ingredients

¼ cup brown sugar
2 tablespoons sea salt
1 tablespoon onion powder
1 tablespoon garlic powder
1 ½ teaspoons ground cumin
2 tablespoons paprika
2 tablespoons ground black pepper
1 ½ teaspoons dried sage
1 pinch crushed red pepper
1 pinch dried thyme
1 pinch chili powder

Directions

1

Mix brown sugar, sea salt, paprika, black pepper, onion powder, garlic powder, cumin, sage, red pepper flakes, chili powder, and thyme in a bowl until well blended. Store in an airtight container.

Nutrition
Per Serving:

18 calories; protein 0.3g; carbohydrates 4.2g; fat 0.2g; sodium 530.4mg.

Pork Stir Fry

Prep:

45 mins

Cook:

15 mins

Total:

1 hr

Servings:

4

Yield:

4 servings

Ingredients

2 tablespoons soy sauce

1 tablespoon cornstarch

¼ cup chopped green onions

1 lime, juiced

1 tablespoon soy sauce

2 tablespoons rice vinegar

1 teaspoon cornstarch

1 tablespoon water

1 pound pork tenderloin, cubed

3 teaspoons dark sesame oil

1 tablespoon peanut oil

2 green chile peppers, chopped

½ cup julienned carrots

½ cup sugar snap peas, julienned

3 teaspoons minced fresh ginger root

2 teaspoons chili oil

¼ cup finely chopped peanuts

Directions

1

In a medium bowl, combine 2 tablespoons soy sauce, 1 tablespoon cornstarch and water. Mix all together until smooth and stir in the pork cubes. Cover and refrigerate for 30 to 45 minutes.

2

In a small bowl combine the lime juice, 1 tablespoon soy sauce, vinegar, 1 teaspoon cornstarch and sesame oil. Mix together and set aside.

3

Remove pork and marinade from refrigerator. In a large skillet or wok heat peanut oil until hot. Stir in ginger and chile pepper and saute for 1 minute. Then stir in pork with marinade, carrots, and sugar peas and stir-fry about 8 minutes or until pork is tender.

4

Pour in lime mixture, reduce heat and simmer until sauce thickens, about 7 minutes. Remove from heat and stir in hot chile oil, green onions and peanuts. Serve!

Nutrition
Per Serving:

318 calories; protein 27.7g; carbohydrates 13.3g; fat 17.5g; cholesterol 73.7mg; sodium 750mg.

Pesto Pasta

Prep:

5 mins

Cook:

20 mins

Total:

25 mins

Servings:

6

Yield:

6 servings

Ingredients

1 pound uncooked pasta
1 (15 ounce) can Del Monte® Sweet Peas, drained
1 Chopped fresh tomatoes
1 cup packed fresh spinach leaves
⅓ cup grated Parmesan cheese, plus more for optional topping
¼ cup olive oil
1 cup packed fresh basil leaves
¼ cup chopped walnuts
¼ teaspoon salt
¼ teaspoon ground black pepper
2 cloves garlic, peeled

Directions

1

Cook pasta according to package directions.

2

Meanwhile, place peas, spinach, basil, Parmesan, olive oil, walnuts, garlic and salt and pepper in a blender or food processor.

3

Two minutes before pasta is done, ladle out 1/2 cup hot pasta cooking water and add to blender. Pulse until smooth, scraping sides and adding additional pasta water by the tablespoon, if needed.

4

When pasta is done, drain lightly and return to pot. Add sauce and toss to coat. Season to taste with salt and pepper. Serve immediately with additional Parmesan cheese and tomatoes, if desired.

Nutrition
Per Serving:

454 calories; protein 14.7g; carbohydrates 66.4g; fat 14.7g; cholesterol 3.9mg; sodium 396.5mg.

Caprese Fusilli

Prep:
35 mins
Total:
35 mins
Servings:
2
Yield:
2 servings

Ingredients

1 (7.75 ounce) package DOLE® Extra Veggie™ with Grape Tomatoes
1 pinch Salt and ground black pepper, to taste
1 clove garlic, minced
2 links hot Italian sausage, cooked and chopped in bite-size pieces
1 cup dry fusilli pasta or rotini pasta, cooked according to package directions
1 tablespoon olive oil
¼ cup chicken broth
Grated Parmesan cheese

Directions
1
Remove grape tomatoes from pouch and cut in half; set aside.

2
Saute garlic and cooked sausage in olive oil in large skillet over medium-high heat 2 to 3 minutes or until garlic is

softened. Add salad blend and tomatoes; saute 3 to 4 minutes longer or until salad blend starts to wilt.

3

Add cooked pasta and broth; cook, stirring until heated through. Season with salt and pepper, to taste. Sprinkle with Parmesan cheese.

Nutrition
Per Serving:

475 calories; protein 24.5g; carbohydrates 26.3g; fat 30.2g; cholesterol 69.3mg; sodium 895.1mg.

Red Wine Risotto

Prep:

10 mins

Cook:

30 mins

Total:

40 mins

Servings:

4

Yield:

4 servings

Ingredients

2 tablespoons olive oil

1 ½ ounces prosciutto

1 large shallot, minced

2 chanterelle mushrooms, sliced

1 cup arborio rice

1 cup red wine

1 clove garlic, chopped

3 cups beef stock, or more as needed, divided

½ cup arugula

1 tablespoon chopped fresh thyme

ground black pepper to taste

⅓ cup freshly grated Parmesan cheese

Directions

1

Heat olive oil in a Dutch oven or heavy pot over medium heat; cook prosciutto until edges begin to curl and fat is rendered, 2 to 3 minutes. Add shallot and cook until fragrant, about 2 minutes. Add garlic and cook until fragrant, about 1 minute. Add mushrooms and cook for 30 seconds.

2

Cook and stir rice into prosciutto mixture, stirring continually, until rice is translucent around edges, 1 to 2 minutes. Pour red wine into rice mixture; cook, stirring every 30 seconds, until wine is absorbed, about 5 minutes. Stir 1 cup broth into rice mixture, cooking and stirring until broth is almost completely absorbed, 4-5 minutes. Continue adding 1 cup broth at a time, stirring constantly, until rice is tender, 15 to 20 minutes.

3

Mix arugula, Parmesan cheese, thyme, and black pepper into rice mixture; cook and stir until cheese is melted, 2 to 4 minutes.

Nutrition

Per Serving:

408 calories; protein 11.8g; carbohydrates 48.7g; fat 12.9g; cholesterol 15.2mg; sodium 380.5mg.

Carrot Noodles

Prep:

15 mins

Cook:

20 mins

Total:

35 mins

Servings:

3

Yield:

3 servings

Ingredients

1 pound carrots
3 tablespoons unsalted butter
¼ pound sliced ham, cut into thin strips
2 cloves garlic, minced
½ cup dry white wine
½ cup minced onion
1 cup heavy cream
salt and pepper to taste
1 cup frozen peas, thawed
1 tablespoon Dijon mustard

Directions

1

Use a vegetable peeler to shave carrots into fettucine-like strands.

2

Heat butter in a large skillet over medium-high heat; when foam subsides, add onion and ham. Cook and stir for 3 minutes.

3

Add carrot strands, garlic, and wine to the skillet with the onion mixture. Reduce heat to low and cover. Cook, stirring occasionally, about 10 minutes.

4

Add cream and peas to the skillet. Bring the mixture to a boil. Reduce heat, cover, and simmer 5 minutes more. Stir in mustard, salt, and pepper.

Nutrition
Per Serving:

591 calories; protein 12.5g; carbohydrates 30.4g; fat 44.7g; cholesterol 160.8mg; sodium 866.1mg.

Shrimp and Asparagus Risotto

Prep:

20 mins

Cook:

32 mins

Total:

52 mins

Servings:

4

Yield:

4 servings

Ingredients

1 (32 ounce) container chicken broth
2 tablespoons olive oil
½ clove garlic, minced
3 cups Arborio rice
1 pound raw shrimp, peeled and deveined
1 pound fresh asparagus, cut into thirds
⅓ onion, chopped
½ cup grated Parmesan cheese
1 tablespoon ground black pepper
1 tablespoon chopped fresh parsley
3 tablespoons butter
1 tablespoon salt

Directions

1

Pour chicken broth into a pot; bring to a simmer over medium-low heat.

2

Heat olive oil in a large saucepan over medium heat. Cook and stir onion and garlic in the hot oil until slightly softened, about 2 minutes. Add Arborio rice; cook, stirring frequently, until coated with oil, about 4 minutes.

3

Stir 1/2 cup of the hot chicken broth into the saucepan; cook and stir until the rice has absorbed the broth, about 2 minutes. Repeat this process 4 more times, stirring constantly, until rice is creamy and tender yet firm to the bite, about 15 minutes.

4

Stir shrimp and asparagus into the remaining hot broth. Cook until shrimp turns pink, 2 to 4 minutes. Remove broth from heat.

5

Stir shrimp and asparagus into the rice; cook for 1 minute. Stir Parmesan cheese and butter into the rice; cook until melted, about 1 minute. Remove rice from heat. Season with salt and pepper. Sprinkle parsley over each serving.

Baked Spaghetti

Prep:

25 mins

Cook:

1 hr

Total:

1 hr 25 mins

Servings:

8

Yield:

8 servings

Ingredients

1 (16 ounce) package spaghetti
1 (32 ounce) jar meatless spaghetti sauce
½ teaspoon seasoned salt
2 eggs
⅓ cup grated Parmesan cheese
1 pound ground beef
1 onion, chopped
5 tablespoons butter, melted
2 cups small curd cottage cheese, divided
4 cups shredded mozzarella cheese, divided

Directions

1

Preheat oven to 350 degrees F. Lightly grease a 9x13-inch baking dish.

2

Bring a large pot of lightly salted water to a boil. Cook spaghetti in boiling water, stirring occasionally until cooked through but firm to the bite, about 10 minutes. Drain.

3

Heat a large skillet over medium heat; cook and stir beef and onion until meat is browned and onions are soft and translucent, about 8 minutes. Drain. Stir in spaghetti sauce and seasoned salt.

4

Whisk eggs, Parmesan cheese, and butter in a large bowl. Mix in spaghetti to egg mixture and toss to coat. Place half the spaghetti mixture into baking dish. Top with half the cottage cheese, mozzarella, and meat sauce. Repeat layers. Cover with aluminum foil.

5

Bake in preheated oven for 40 minutes. Remove foil and continue to bake until the cheese is melted and lightly browned, 20 to 25 minutes longer.

Nutrition
Per Serving:

728 calories; protein 42.5g; carbohydrates 61.9g; fat 33.6g; cholesterol 150.2mg; sodium 1250.5mg.

Squash Linguine

Prep:

20 mins

Cook:

5 mins

Total:

25 mins

Servings:

4

Yield:

4 servings

Ingredients

¼ cup extra-virgin olive oil
1 (8 ounce) container skim milk ricotta cheese, divided
2 tablespoons minced garlic
salt and ground black pepper to taste
1 large zucchini, sliced into thin rounds
1 large yellow squash, sliced into thin rounds
½ cup chopped fresh basil
½ cup chopped fresh basil
1 cup cherry or grape tomatoes, halved
1 (16 ounce) package fresh linguine pasta

Directions

1

Whisk olive oil, garlic, 1/2 cup of basil, salt, and pepper in a large bowl. Add zucchini, yellow squash, and tomatoes to the oil mixture and toss to coat.

2

Bring a large pot of lightly salted water to a boil. Cook the linguine at a boil until tender yet firm to the bite, about 6 to 9 minutes; drain. Transfer pasta to a serving bowl.

3

While the pasta is warm, fold in half of vegetable mixture along with 2 tablespoons ricotta cheese, until pasta is coated and vegetables are evenly dispersed. Top with remaining vegetable mixture. Spoon remaining ricotta on top. Sprinkle 1/2 cup chopped basil over the dish. Season with salt and pepper to serve.

Nutrition
Per Serving:

610 calories; protein 20.8g; carbohydrates 92.6g; fat 16.4g; cholesterol 10mg; sodium 81.4mg.

Ratatouille

Prep:

15 mins

Cook:

1 hr 5 mins

Total:

1 hr 20 mins

Servings:

6

Yield:

6 servings

Ingredients

½ cup extra-virgin olive oil

2 pounds fresh tomatoes, quartered

2 large onions, quartered

3 tablespoons herbes de Provence

salt and ground black pepper to taste

3 cloves garlic, minced

3 eggplants, sliced into 1/2-inch rounds

6 zucchini, sliced 1/2-inch thick

Directions

1

Pour olive oil into a large pot over high heat. Add onions and garlic and saute for 2 minutes. Reduce heat and add tomatoes, eggplants, zucchini, tomato puree, herbes de Provence, salt, and pepper. Cover and simmer for 30 minutes.

2

Uncover and check the level of liquid in the pot. Continue cooking for 30 minutes, uncovered if there is too much liquid, or covered if the amount of liquid looks right.

Nutrition
Per Serving:

323 calories; protein 7.5g; carbohydrates 35.2g; fat 19.9g; sodium 143.9mg.

Zucchini Crisp

Prep:

15 mins

Cook:

45 mins

Total:

1 hr

Servings:

20

Yield:

1 9x13-inch crisp

Ingredients

8 cups cubed peeled zucchini

½ cup white sugar

⅓ cup lemon juice

1 teaspoon ground nutmeg

1 cup brown sugar, packed

2 teaspoons ground cinnamon

1 cup rolled oats

½ cup margarine

1 cup all-purpose flour

Directions

1

Preheat oven to 375 degrees F. Grease a 9x13-inch baking dish.

2

Mix zucchini, white sugar, lemon juice, cinnamon, and nutmeg in a large bowl. Pour mixture into baking dish.

3

Combine brown sugar, oats, and flour in another bowl. Cut in margarine until mixture resembles coarse crumbs; sprinkle over zucchini.

4

Bake in preheated oven until bubbly and zucchini is tender, 40 to 45 minutes.

Nutrition
Per Serving:

150 calories; protein 1.9g; carbohydrates 25.6g; fat 5g; sodium 61.1mg.

Zoodles

Prep:

10 mins

Cook:

10 mins

Total:

20 mins

Servings:

2

Yield:

2 servings

Ingredients

1 tablespoon olive oil

½ cup drained and rinsed canned garbanzo beans (chickpeas)

3 tablespoons pesto, or to taste

2 tablespoons shredded white Cheddar cheese

4 small zucchini, cut into noodle-shape strands

salt and ground black pepper to taste

Directions

1

Heat olive oil in a skillet over medium heat; cook and stir zucchini until tender and liquid has evaporated, 6 to 10 minutes.

2

Stir garbanzo beans and pesto into zucchini; lower heat to medium-low. Cook and stir until garbanzo beans are warm and zucchini is evenly coated, about 5 minutes; season with salt and pepper.

3

Transfer zucchini mixture to serving bowls and top with white Cheddar cheese.

Nutrition
Per Serving:

319 calories; protein 12.1g; carbohydrates 23.1g; fat 21.3g; cholesterol 16.2mg; sodium 510.8mg.

Veggie Chili

Prep:

10 mins

Cook:

20 mins

Total:

30 mins

Servings:

8

Yield:

8 servings

Ingredients

1 tablespoon Spectrum® Olive Oil Extra Virgin Cold Pressed

1 ½ cups chopped red onions

1 cup chopped celery

2 teaspoons minced garlic

1 (340 gram) package Yves Veggie Cuisine® Mexican Veggie Ground Round

1 ½ tablespoons chili powder

1 cup chopped green bell pepper

2 teaspoons ground cumin

2 teaspoons dried oregano

½ teaspoon crushed red pepper flakes

¼ teaspoon ground cinnamon

1 (796 mL) can diced tomatoes, undrained

1 teaspoon ground coriander

2 (540 mL) cans Yves Veggie Cuisine® Organic Black Beans, canned

1 cup Imagine® Organic Vegetable Broth

1 tablespoon brown sugar

1 (398 mL) can tomato sauce

½ teaspoon salt

¼ teaspoon freshly ground black pepper

Directions

1

Heat olive oil in a large, non-stick pot over medium-high heat.

2

Add onions, green pepper, celery and garlic. Cook and stir until vegetables begin to soften, about 5 minutes.

3

Add Yves Veggie Ground Round, chili powder, cumin, oregano, coriander, red pepper flakes and cinnamon. Mix well and cook for 1 more minute.

4

Add undrained tomatoes, beans, tomato sauce, broth, brown sugar, salt and pepper. Bring mixture to a boil. Reduce heat to low and simmer, covered for 20 minutes.

5

Remove from heat and stir in cilantro (if using). Serve hot.

Nutrition

Per Serving:

281 calories; protein 18.5g; carbohydrates 42.6g; fat 4.8g; sodium 1039.1mg.

Roasted Vegetables

Prep:

30 mins

Cook:

20 mins

Total:

50 mins

Servings:

8

Yield:

8 servings

Ingredients

5 cups cauliflower florets

1 pound fresh asparagus, trimmed and halved

4 medium carrots, cut into matchsticks

1 medium red bell pepper, cut into matchsticks

½ cup olive oil

3 tablespoons lemon juice

3 cloves garlic, minced

1 medium red onion, sliced and separated into rings

1 teaspoon salt

5 cups broccoli florets

1 teaspoon ground black pepper

1 tablespoon dried rosemary, crushed

Directions

1

Preheat the oven to 400 degrees F.

2

Combine cauliflower, broccoli, asparagus, carrots, bell pepper, and onion in a large bowl.

3

Whisk olive oil, lemon juice, garlic, rosemary, salt, and pepper together in a small bowl until blended. Drizzle over vegetables and toss to coat. Transfer to 2 rimmed baking sheets.

4

Roast in the preheated oven, tossing occasionally, until tender, 20 to 25 minutes.

Nutrition
Per Serving:

194 calories; protein 4.8g; carbohydrates 15.7g; fat 14.1g; sodium 352.6mg.

Mushroom Tacos

Prep:
30 mins
Cook:
10 mins
Total:
40 mins
Servings:
8
Yield:
8 tacos

Ingredients

4 tablespoons olive oil
¼ cup crumbled blue cheese, or to taste
1 ½ cups chopped onion
3 cloves garlic, minced
8 corn tortillas
1 pound ground venison
1 package taco seasoning
1 cup shredded cabbage
2 tablespoons lime juice
2 tablespoons chopped cilantro
salt and ground black pepper to taste
1 (8 ounce) jar salsa
1 (8 ounce) package mushrooms, finely chopped or pulsed in a food processor

Directions

1

Heat olive oil in a saute pan over medium-high heat. Add onions and cook about 3 minutes. Add garlic and cook 2 minutes more. Add venison and mushrooms; saute until venison is cooked through, 6 to 7 minutes more. Season with taco seasoning.

2

Toss cabbage, lime juice, cilantro, salt, and pepper together in a bowl.

3

Place about 2 tablespoons cabbage mixture onto a tortilla and top with about 2 tablespoons meat mixture. Top with salsa and blue cheese. Repeat with remaining fillings, tortillas, and toppings.

Nutrition

Per Serving:

238 calories; protein 15.8g; carbohydrates 21.5g; fat 10.1g; cholesterol 45.9mg; sodium 596.2mg

Italian Orecchiette

Prep:

15 mins

Cook:

30 mins

Total:

45 mins

Servings:

6

Yield:

6 servings

Ingredients

12 ounces orecchiette pasta

1 tablespoon olive oil

1 teaspoon Italian seasoning

freshly ground black pepper to taste

1 pound ground Italian sausage

¼ cup diced green bell pepper

½ cup diced green onion

2 cloves garlic, minced

½ cup butter

1 ½ cups half-and-half

6 ounces freshly grated Parmesan cheese

1 bunch broccolini, sliced into 1-inch pieces

4 ounces cream cheese

1 teaspoon salt

Directions

1

Bring a large pot of salted water to a boil. Add 1 tablespoon olive oil and orecchiette and cook, stirring occasionally, until tender yet firm to the bite, 8 to 10 minutes. Drain and set aside.

2

Meanwhile, heat a large skillet over medium-high heat. Cook and stir sausage in the hot skillet until browned and crumbly, 6 to 7 minutes. Drain and discard most of the fat. Transfer cooked sausage to a bowl and return skillet to medium-high heat.

3

Add bell pepper and green onion to the skillet. Saute until white of onion becomes translucent, about 5 minutes. Add broccolini and garlic; saute until broccolini is crisp-tender, about 3 minutes more. Set vegetables aside.

4

Melt butter in a larger skillet over medium heat. Add half-and-half and Parmesan cheese, stirring constantly until bubbly, about 5 minutes. Add cream cheese, Italian seasoning, salt, and pepper. Cook until sauce begins to thicken, about 5 minutes more.

5

Add cooked sausage and vegetables to the skillet. Stir in drained pasta. Serve immediately.

Nutrition

Per Serving:

840 calories; protein 34.2g; carbohydrates 54.3g; fat 54.6g; cholesterol 138.5mg; sodium 1664.5mg.

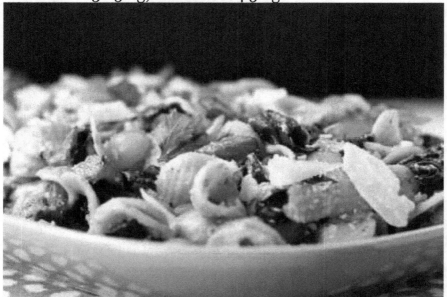

Tuna Steaks

Prep:

5 mins

Cook:

6 mins

Total:

11 mins

Servings:

4

Yield:

4 servings

Ingredients

2 tablespoons olive oil

2 tablespoons grated lemon zest

½ teaspoon ground cinnamon

4 (5 ounce) tuna steaks, about 1 inch thick

1 ¼ teaspoons ground black pepper

1 ½ teaspoons ground ginger

1 teaspoon salt

1 tablespoon olive oil

2 teaspoons ground coriander

Directions

1

Whisk 2 tablespoons olive oil, lemon zest, coriander, black pepper, ginger, salt, and cinnamon in a small bowl; rub tuna steaks with spice mixture.

2

Heat 1 tablespoon olive oil in a large skillet over medium-high heat. Sear tuna in the hot oil until browned but still pink in the center, about 3 minutes on each side.

Nutrition
Per Serving:

254 calories; protein 33.4g; carbohydrates 2.2g; fat 11.7g; cholesterol 64.1mg; sodium 634.5mg.

Salmon Fillet

Prep:

10 mins

Cook:

15 mins

Total:

25 mins

Servings:

4

Yield:

1 pound salmon

Ingredients

2 tablespoons miso paste

2 tablespoons mirin (Japanese sweet wine)

1 tablespoon soy sauce

1 teaspoon honey

1 tablespoon oil

1 pound salmon fillets

1 tablespoon minced ginger

1 teaspoon sesame seeds

Directions

1

Toast sesame seeds in a small saucepan over medium heat, stirring occasionally, about 2 minutes. Watch them closely and remove from heat once sesame seeds are a golden brown. Set aside.

2

Combine miso paste, mirin, soy sauce, ginger, and honey in a small bowl. Mix well. Stir in toasted sesame seeds.

3

Set an oven rack about 6 inches from the heat source and preheat the oven's broiler. Line a baking pan with foil and lightly grease with oil.

4

Coat salmon well in the miso sauce and place skin-side up on the baking pan.

5

Broil in the preheated oven, watching closely, until fish flakes easily with a fork, 10 to 14 minutes.

Nutrition

Per Serving:

240 calories; protein 25.7g; carbohydrates 6.9g; fat 11g; cholesterol 50.4mg; sodium 595.8mg.

Pantry Puttanesca

Prep:

5 mins

Cook:

16 mins

Total:

21 mins

Servings:

4

Yield:

4 servings

Ingredients

⅓ cup olive oil

3 cloves garlic, minced

½ cup chopped pitted kalamata olives

1 teaspoon dried oregano

3 anchovy fillets, chopped

2 (15 ounce) cans diced tomatoes, drained.

1 (8 ounce) package spaghetti

¼ cup capers, chopped

¼ teaspoon crushed red pepper flakes

Directions

1

Fill a large pot with water. Bring to a rolling boil over high heat.

2

As the water heats, pour the olive oil into a cold skillet and stir in the garlic. Turn heat to medium-low and cook and stir until the garlic is fragrant and begins to turn a golden color, 1 to 2 minutes. Stir in the red pepper flakes, oregano, and anchovies. Cook until anchovies begin to break down, about 2 minutes.

3

Pour tomatoes into skillet, turn heat to medium-high, and bring sauce to a simmer. Use the back of a spoon to break down tomatoes as they cook. Simmer until sauce is reduced and combined, about 10-12 minutes.

4

Meanwhile, cook the pasta in the boiling water. Drain when still very firm to the bite, about 10 minutes. Reserve 1/2 cup pasta water.

5

Stir the olives and capers into the sauce; add pasta and toss to combine.

6

Toss pasta in sauce until pasta is cooked through and well coated with sauce, about 1 minute. If sauce becomes too thick, stir in some of the reserved pasta water to thin.

Nutrition
Per Serving:

463 calories; protein 10.5g; carbohydrates 53.3g; fat 24g; cholesterol 2.5mg; sodium 944.5mg.

Salmon Fillets with Dill

Prep:

15 mins

Cook:

15 mins

Total:

30 mins

Servings:

4

Yield:

4 servings

Ingredients

4 (6 ounce) fillets salmon

½ cup water

3 lemon slices, cut into quarters

⅓ cup lemon juice

1 ½ teaspoons cornstarch

2 lemons, ends trimmed and sliced thickly

4 teaspoons butter

1 tablespoon snipped fresh dill

¼ teaspoon salt

1 dash cayenne pepper

⅛ teaspoon dried chervil

Directions

1

Preheat an outdoor grill for high heat and lightly oil the grate.

2

Grill salmon and thick lemon slices on hot grill until salmon flakes easily with a fork, 3 to 5 minutes per side.

3

Stir water, lemon juice, and cornstarch together in a small saucepan to dissolve the cornstarch; add butter and place over medium heat. Cook and stir the mixture until boiling and thick, 5 to 10 minutes. Remove saucepan from heat. Stir quartered lemon slices, dill, salt, chervil, and cayenne pepper into the sauce. Serve with the grilled salmon and grilled lemon slices.

Nutrition
Per Serving:

243 calories; protein 33.8g; carbohydrates 4g; fat 9.9g; cholesterol 98.5mg; sodium 288.9mg.

Herb Potatoes

Prep:

5 mins

Cook:

40 mins

Total:

45 mins

Servings:

5

Yield:

4 to 6 servings

Ingredients

2 tablespoons olive oil

3 large carrots, sliced diagonally

1 tablespoon balsamic vinegar

1 teaspoon garlic salt

¼ teaspoon ground black pepper

2 small Vidalia onions, wedged

1 teaspoon dried rosemary, crushed

2 red potatoes, chopped

Directions

1

Heat a barbeque to a high heat, or preheat oven to 400 degrees F.

2

In a 9x13 inch baking dish combine olive oil, vinegar, garlic salt, rosemary, and ground black pepper. Place carrots, potatoes, and onions into the dish and toss to coat.

3

Bake or grill, turning occasionally, until tender (approximately 40 minutes).

Nutrition

Per Serving:

153 calories; protein 2.7g; carbohydrates 23.7g; fat 5.7g; sodium 385.6mg.

Blistered Tomatoes

Prep:

10 mins

Cook:

40 mins

Total:

50 mins

Servings:

4

Yield:

4 servings

Ingredients

2 pints whole cherry tomatoes
6 sprigs fresh thyme, leaves removed
6 sprigs fresh oregano, leaves removed
½ cup fresh sage leaves
½ cup olive oil
Reynolds Wrap® Aluminum Foil
Salt and cracked black pepper to taste

Directions

1

Preheat oven to 400 degrees F. Line a rimmed baking sheet with Reynolds Wrap® Aluminum Foil. Place cherry tomatoes on the prepared baking sheet.

2

Distribute sage and thyme amongst tomatoes, reserving about 1 tablespoon of each for garnishing. Drizzle generously with olive oil. Sprinkle with salt and pepper. Roast for 30 minutes or until tomatoes blister.

3

Remove tomatoes and place into a bowl, tossing all juices collected in the foil. Garnish with additional fresh thyme, sage and oregano. Season with salt and pepper to taste and serve.

Nutrition
Per Serving:

278 calories; protein 1.5g; carbohydrates 8g; fat 27.8g; sodium 53mg.

Fish Soup

Prep:

10 mins

Cook:

30 mins

Total:

40 mins

Servings:

4

Yield:

4 servings

Ingredients

½ onion, chopped
¾ cup plain nonfat yogurt
1 clove garlic, minced
1 ½ cups chicken broth
1 (4 ounce) can canned green chile peppers, chopped
1 teaspoon ground cumin
1 tablespoon chili powder
½ cup chopped green bell pepper
½ cup shrimp
1 ½ cups canned peeled and diced tomatoes
½ pound cod fillets

Directions

1

Spray a large saucepan with the vegetable cooking spray over medium high heat. Add the onions and saute, stirring often, for about 5 minutes. Add the garlic and chili powder and saute for 2 more minutes.

2

Then add the chicken broth, chile peppers and cumin, stirring well. Bring to a boil, reduce heat to low, cover and simmer for 20 minutes.

3

Next, add the tomatoes, green bell pepper, shrimp and cod. Return to a boil, then reduce heat to low, cover and simmer for another 5 minutes. Gradually stir in the yogurt until heated through.

Nutrition

Per Serving:

146 calories; protein 19.3g; carbohydrates 12.2g; fat 1.7g; cholesterol 45.7mg; sodium 873.8mg.

CHAPTER 3: DINNER

Samosas in Potatoes

Prep:

45 mins

Cook:

20 mins

Additional:

30 mins

Total:

1 hr 35 mins

Servings:

10

Yield:

20 samosas

Ingredients

1/8 teaspoon cayenne pepper

1 1/2 pounds russet potatoes, peeled and diced

1/2 teaspoon ground turmeric

1/2 cup frozen peas

1 teaspoon garam masala

1 teaspoon salt

Dough:

1 1/2 cups all-purpose flour

3/4 teaspoon salt

1 tablespoon vegetable oil

6 tablespoons ice water, or more if needed

Filling:
¼ cup butter
4 teaspoons ginger-garlic paste
1 tablespoon olive oil
½ cup chopped yellow onion
1 cup vegetable oil for frying
1 squeeze lemon juice

Directions

1

Place potatoes into a large pot and cover with salted water; bring to a boil. Reduce heat to medium-low and simmer until just tender, about 10 minutes.

2

Meanwhile, place peas in a microwave-safe bowl and cook in the microwave until heated through, 2 to 3 minutes. Set aside. Combine garam masala, salt, turmeric, and cayenne pepper in a bowl and set spice mixture aside.

3

Mix flour and salt together in a bowl. Drizzle in oil and rub in using your fingers. Add about 6 tablespoons ice water and work it into the dough. Add additional ice water as necessary to create a firm dough. Knead for 1 to 2 minutes and put aside to rest for 30 minutes.

4

Meanwhile, drain potatoes. Heat butter and oil in a large frying pan. Add onion and ginger-garlic paste; cook and stir until onions are translucent and beginning to brown, 5 to 10 minutes. Add spice mixture and stir to combine. Add cooked potatoes and stir. Mash using a fork or potato masher to the desired consistency. Add cooked peas and lemon juice; mix filling until well combined.

5

Knead dough and tear off approximately 10 equal-sized pieces. Roll each piece into a ball and roll each ball into a thin circle about 6 inches in diameter. Cut dough circles in half. Add a spoon of filling to each half-circle; use a finger dipped in water to wet the edges of the dough and press edges together using a fork to seal.

6

Heat oil in a large frying pan over medium-high heat. Fry samosas in the hot oil until golden brown, about 4 minutes each.

Nutrition

Per Serving: 220 calories; protein 3.9g; carbohydrates 28.2g; fat 9.9g; cholesterol 12.2mg; sodium 521.9mg.

Classic Socca

Prep:

10 mins

Cook:

20 mins

Additional:

2 hrs

Total:

2 hrs 30 mins

Servings:

4

Yield:

2 flatbreads

Ingredients

1 cup chickpea flour
salt and ground black pepper to taste
1 cup water
½ teaspoon ground cumin
1 tablespoon vegetable oil for frying
1 tablespoon olive oil

Directions

1

Combine chickpea flour, water, and olive oil in a bowl. Season with cumin, salt, and pepper to taste. Stir everything together until smooth. Set aside and let rest at room temperature for 2 hours.

2

Preheat the oven to 450 degrees F. Place a cast iron skillet in the oven until hot, about 6 minutes.

3

Carefully remove skillet from oven, grease with oil and pour half of the the batter into the skillet, tilting so batter is evenly distributed.

4

Bake in the preheated oven until socca is set, about 7-8 minutes. Turn on broiler and brown for 1 minute. Remove from oven and slide onto a plate. Repeat with remaining batter.

Nutrition

Per Serving: 146 calories; protein 4.7g; carbohydrates 13.8g; fat 8.4g; sodium 41mg.

Ritzy Garden Burgers

Prep:

20 mins

Cook:

30 mins

Total:

50 mins

Servings:

2

Yield:

2 servings

Ingredients

1 (8 ounce) package buttery round crackers

¾ cup freshly grated Parmesan cheese

1 teaspoon onion powder

1 teaspoon black pepper

1 teaspoon salt

2 eggs, beaten

½ lime, juiced

1 teaspoon garlic powder

1 eggplant, peeled and sliced into 1/2 inch rounds

Directions

1

Preheat oven to 375 degrees F. Spray baking sheet with cooking spray or lightly grease with olive oil.

2

Crumble crackers into a large bowl. Stir in onion powder, black pepper, garlic powder, and salt.

3

In a separate bowl, stir together eggs and lime juice.

4

Dip eggplant slices into egg mixture, then dredge in cracker mix, and place on baking sheet.

5

Bake in preheated oven for 15 minutes. Turn eggplant pieces, top with grated cheese, and cook an additional 15 minutes.

Nutrition

Per Serving: 880 calories; protein 30.2g; carbohydrates 84.4g; fat 47.6g; cholesterol 219mg; sodium 2838.2mg.

Za'atar Bread

Prep:

30 mins

Cook:

25 mins

Total:

55 mins

Servings:

40

Yield:

40 servings

Ingredients

3 cups warm water
2 cups fresh za'atar
1 (.25 ounce) package yeast
2 cups whole wheat flour
1 teaspoon salt
1 teaspoon white sugar
8 cups all-purpose flour
2 cups olive oil
1 cup corn oil

Directions

1

Preheat oven to 350 degrees F.

2

Mix water, yeast, salt, and sugar together in a large bowl. Add all-purpose flour, whole wheat flour, olive oil, and corn oil;

mix using your hands, adding more whole wheat flour if needed, until dough holds together. Mix za'atar into dough until evenly incorporated.

3
Shape dough, about 1/4 cup per piece, into rounds on a floured work surface. Arrange rounds on baking sheets.

4
Bake in the preheated oven until lightly browned, about 25-27 minutes.

Nutrition
Per Serving: 266 calories; protein 3.8g; carbohydrates 25.8g; fat 16.9g; sodium 61.7mg.

Slaw

Prep:

15 mins

Cook:

5 mins

Total:

20 mins

Servings:

8

Yield:

8 servings

Ingredients

¼ cup chopped pecans

1 tablespoon sugar

1 (8.5 ounce) package coleslaw mix

¼ cup crumbled feta cheese

½ cup mayonnaise

½ cup Ranch dressing

½ cup matchstick-style shredded carrots

1 ½ cups red grapes

Directions

1

In a medium ungreased skillet, over medium heat, toast the pecans by stirring frequently until golden brown. Set aside to cool.

2

In a large bowl, combine coleslaw mix, carrots, grapes, pecans, and feta cheese.

3

In a small bowl, stir together the mayonnaise, and Ranch dressing. Pour in sugar, and mix until dissolved. Toss coleslaw mixture with dressing until evenly coated. Serve immediately.

Nutrition

Per Serving: 265 calories; protein 2g; carbohydrates 13.2g; fat 23.4g; cholesterol 15.9mg; sodium 286.8mg.

Pizza Pockets

Cook:

15 mins

Additional:

10 mins

Total:

25 mins

Servings:

4

Yield:

4 servings

Ingredients

¼ cup pizza sauce

½ cup sliced pepperoni

1 teaspoon grated Parmesan cheese

¾ cup shredded mozzarella cheese

1 (8 ounce) can Pillsbury® refrigerated crescent dinner rolls

Directions

1

Heat oven to 375 degrees F. Unroll dough on cookie sheet and separate into 4 rectangles; press each into 6x4-inch rectangle, firmly pressing perforations to seal.

2

Spread 1 tablespoon pizza sauce on half of each rectangle to within 1 inch of edge. Sprinkle each with 3 tablespoons cheese; top with 6 slices pepperoni. Fold dough diagonally over filling; firmly press edges with fork to seal. Sprinkle each triangle with 1/4 teaspoon grated cheese. With fork, prick top of each to allow steam to escape.

3

Bake 13 to 16 minutes or until deep golden brown. Serve warm.

Nutrition

Per Serving: 426 calories; protein 16.1g; carbohydrates 24.3g; fat 28.2g; cholesterol 43.8mg; sodium 1135.5mg.

Brown Rice

Prep:

5 mins

Cook:

1 hr

Total:

1 hr 5 mins

Servings:

4

Yield:

4 to 6 servings

Ingredients

1 (14 ounce) can beef broth

1 tablespoon dried basil leaves

1 (10.5 ounce) can condensed French onion soup

¼ cup butter, melted

1 ½ cups uncooked long-grain white rice

1 tablespoon Worcestershire sauce

Directions

1

Preheat oven to 350 degrees F.

2

In a 2 quart casserole dish combine rice, broth, soup, butter, Worcestershire sauce and basil.

3

Bake covered for 1 hour, stirring once after 30 minutes.

Nutrition

Per Serving: 425 calories; protein 8.8g; carbohydrates 66.2g; fat 13.5g; cholesterol 33.4mg; sodium 1091mg.

Cauliflower and Broccoli Bowls

Prep:

15 mins

Cook:

30 mins

Total:

45 mins

Servings:

5

Yield:

5 servings

Ingredients

½ cup cashews

½ teaspoon salt

4 cups broccoli florets

4 cups cauliflower florets

½ teaspoon garlic powder

1 (15 ounce) can chickpeas (garbanzo beans), drained and rinsed

2 tablespoons lemon juice

salt and ground black pepper to taste

1 tablespoon tahini

Directions

1

Place cashews in a bowl and top with water; soak until softened, 3 to 4 hours.

2

Preheat oven to 400 degrees F. Line 2 baking sheets with parchment paper or spray with cooking spray.

3

Spread broccoli and cauliflower onto 1 baking sheet and season with garlic powder, salt, and pepper. Spread chickpeas onto the other baking sheet and season with salt and pepper.

4

Roast in the preheated oven until broccoli, cauliflower, and chickpeas are softened and cooked through, about 30 minutes.

5

Drain cashews. Combine cashews, lemon juice, tahini, and 1/2 teaspoon salt in a blender or food processor; blend until dressing is smooth.

6

Transfer broccoli, cauliflower, and chickpeas to serving bowl. Drizzle dressing over vegetables and chickpeas.

Nutrition
Per Serving: 210 calories; protein 9g; carbohydrates 27.4g; fat 8.9g; sodium 569.5mg.

Mahi-Mahi Meal

Prep:

30 mins

Additional:

1 hr

Total:

1 hr 30 mins

Servings:

6

Yield:

6 servings

Ingredients

⅓ cup lime juice

⅓ cup lemon juice

1 tablespoon minced jalapeno pepper

1 pinch dried oregano

1 pinch cayenne pepper

½ cup diced avocados

½ cup peeled and seeded diced cucumber

½ teaspoon salt

½ cup diced orange segments

½ cup chopped fresh chives

¾ pound mahi mahi fillets, diced

1 tablespoon chopped cilantro

1 tablespoon olive oil

2 tablespoons radishes, sliced

Directions

1

Stir mahi mahi, lime juice, lemon juice, jalapeno pepper, salt, oregano, and cayenne pepper together in a bowl. Press down fish to completely immerse in liquid. Cover the bowl with plastic wrap and press plastic wrap down so that it is touching the fish. Refrigerate for at least 1 hour, or up to 6 hours.

2

Stir avocado, cucumber, orange, chives, radish, cilantro, and olive oil into mahi mahi mixture until completely coated. Season with salt.

Nutrition

Per Serving: 117 calories; protein 11.4g; carbohydrates 6.5g; fat 5.6g; cholesterol 41.5mg; sodium 247mg.

Breaded Shrimp

Prep:

5 mins

Cook:

10 mins

Total:

15 mins

Servings:

8

Yield:

8 servings

Ingredients

1 quart vegetable oil for frying

1 egg, beaten

2 cups dry bread crumbs

4 cups shrimp, peeled and deveined

Directions

1

Heat oil in a large skillet. Dip the shrimp in the egg, then coat the shrimp with bread crumbs. Fry the shrimp in the hot oil.

Nutrition

Per Serving: 281 calories; protein 17.4g; carbohydrates 20.1g; fat 14.2g; cholesterol 120.5mg; sodium 301.1mg.

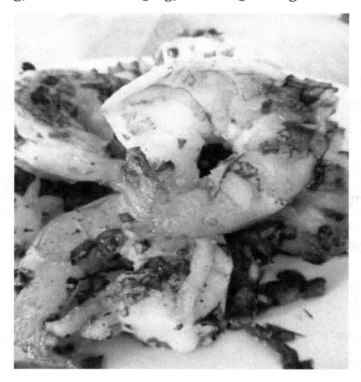

Haddock Marinara

Prep:

15 mins

Cook:

30 mins

Total:

45 mins

Servings:

4

Yield:

4 servings

Ingredients

2 tablespoons extra virgin olive oil

¾ cup shredded mozzarella cheese

½ white onion, finely chopped

3 cloves garlic, minced

1 pound haddock fillets

1 (14 ounce) can stewed tomatoes, drained

1 (16 ounce) jar pasta sauce

Directions

1

Preheat oven to 350 degrees F. Coat the bottom of a baking dish with the olive oil.

2

Sprinkle 1/2 the onion and garlic evenly in the baking dish, and cover with 1/2 the pasta sauce. Place the haddock fillets in the dish, top with tomatoes and remaining onion and garlic. Cover with remaining pasta sauce.

3

Bake 20 minutes in the preheated oven. Top with mozzarella cheese, and continue baking 10 minutes, until cheese is melted and fish is easily flaked with a fork.

Nutrition

Per Serving: 345 calories; protein 29.8g; carbohydrates 24.1g; fat 14.2g; cholesterol 80.5mg; sodium 885mg.

Potato Casserole

Prep:

15 mins

Cook:

1 hr 10 mins

Total:

1 hr 25 mins

Servings:

12

Yield:

6 servings

Ingredients

1 (30 ounce) package frozen hash brown potatoes

1 cup butter

2 cups shredded Cheddar cheese

1 (10.75 ounce) can condensed cream of mushroom soup

1 onion, chopped

1 (16 ounce) container sour cream

3 cups crushed corn flakes

Directions

1

Preheat oven to 425 degrees F.

2

Pour the hash browns into a lightly greased 9x13 inch baking dish. In a large bowl, combine the cheese, sour cream and soup.

3

In a large skillet over medium heat, combine the onion with 1 stick butter and saute for 5 minutes. Add this to the soup mixture and spread this over the potatoes in the dish.

4

Next, arrange the crushed corn flakes over all in the dish. Melt the remaining stick of butter and pour this evenly over the corn flakes.

5

Bake at 425 degrees F for 1 hour.

Nutrition

Per Serving: 400 calories; protein 8.5g; carbohydrates 23.1g; fat 35.5g; cholesterol 77.1mg; sodium 483.4mg.

Crispy Tilapia with Mango Salsa

Prep:

45 mins

Cook:

10 mins

Additional:

1 hr

Total:

1 hr 55 mins

Servings:

2

Yield:

2 servings

Ingredients

⅓ cup extra-virgin olive oil
1 tablespoon lemon juice
2 (6 ounce) tilapia fillets
1 tablespoon minced fresh parsley
1 clove garlic, minced
1 teaspoon dried basil
1 teaspoon ground black pepper
½ teaspoon salt
1 large ripe mango, peeled, pitted and diced
½ red bell pepper, diced
2 tablespoons minced red onion
1 jalapeno pepper, seeded and minced
2 tablespoons lime juice
1 tablespoon lemon juice
1 tablespoon chopped fresh cilantro

salt and pepper to taste

Directions

1

Whisk together the extra-virgin olive oil, 1 tablespoon lemon juice, parsley, garlic, basil, 1 teaspoon pepper, and 1/2 teaspoon salt in a bowl and pour into a resealable plastic bag. Add the tilapia fillets, coat with the marinade, squeeze out excess air, and seal the bag. Marinate in the refrigerator for 1 hour.

2

Prepare the mango salsa by combining the mango, red bell pepper, red onion, cilantro, and jalapeno pepper in a bowl. Add the lime juice and 1 tablespoon of lemon juice, and toss well. Season to taste with salt and pepper, and refrigerate until ready to serve.

3

Preheat an outdoor grill for medium-high heat, and lightly oil grate.

4

Remove the tilapia from the marinade, and shake off excess. Discard the remaining marinade. Grill the fillets until the fish is no longer translucent in the center, and flakes easily with a fork, 3 to 4 minutes per side, depending on the thickness of the fillets. Serve the tilapia topped with mango salsa.

Nutrition

Per Serving: 634 calories; protein 36.3g; carbohydrates 33.4g; fat 40.2g; cholesterol 62.2mg; sodium 696.7mg.

Braised Branzino with Wine Sauce

Prep:

30 mins

Cook:

4 hrs

Total:

4 hrs 30 mins

Servings:

6

Yield:

6 servings

Ingredients

2 (750 milliliter) bottles dry red wine

1 cup all-purpose flour

2 sprigs fresh thyme

1 teaspoon garlic powder

salt and pepper to taste

5 pounds beef oxtail, cut into pieces

¼ cup butter, divided

5 shallots, chopped

5 cloves garlic, chopped

1 teaspoon onion powder

1 onion, chopped

2 carrots, chopped

2 celery ribs, chopped

1 bay leaf

2 sprigs flat-leaf parsley

5 cups beef broth

Directions

1

Preheat oven to 325 degrees F.

2

Simmer the red wine in a large saucepan over medium-high heat until reduced by half. Meanwhile, combine the flour, garlic powder, onion powder, salt, and pepper in a large bowl. Dredge the oxtail in the seasoned flour, and shake off excess; set aside. Heat 1 tablespoon of butter in a roasting pan over medium-high heat. Brown the oxtail on all sides, about 10 minutes.

3

Remove the oxtails from the pan and set aside. Turn the heat to medium-low and melt another 1 tablespoon of butter in the pan. Stir in the shallots, garlic, onion, carrots, and celery. Cook and stir until the vegetables have softened, about 10 minutes. Stir in the thyme, bay leaf, parsley, beef broth, and reduced red wine. Place the browned oxtail on top of the vegetables in a single layer, then bring to a boil.

4

Cover with a tight fitting lid or aluminum foil, then bake in preheated oven until the oxtail is very tender and nearly falling off the bone, 3 to 3 1/2 hours.

5

Once the oxtail is tender, remove the meat to a serving dish, cover, and keep warm. Strain the remaining braising liquid through a mesh strainer into a saucepan. Simmer over medium-high heat until the sauce has reduced to 2 cups. Whisk in the remaining 2 tablespoons butter and pour over the oxtail to serve.

Nutrition

Per Serving: 891 calories; protein 64.6g; carbohydrates 36.4g; fat 33.9g; cholesterol 228.4mg; sodium 1132.4mg.

Peas Soup

Prep:

15 mins

Cook:

2 hrs

Additional:

8 hrs 15 mins

Total:

10 hrs 30 mins

Servings:

6

Yield:

6 to 8 servings

Ingredients

2 ¼ cups dried split peas
1 potato, diced
2 quarts cold water
1 ½ pounds ham bone
½ teaspoon salt
¼ teaspoon ground black pepper
1 pinch dried marjoram
3 stalks celery, chopped
2 onions, thinly sliced
3 carrots, chopped

Directions

1

In a large stock pot, cover peas with 2 quarts cold water and soak overnight. If you need a faster method, simmer the peas gently for 2 minutes, and then soak for 1 hour.

2

Once peas are soaked, add ham bone, onion, salt, pepper and marjoram. Cover, bring to boil and then simmer for 1 1/2 hours, stirring occasionally.

3

Remove bone; cut off meat, dice and return meat to soup. Add celery, carrots and potatoes. Cook slowly, uncovered for 30 to 40 minutes, or until vegetables are tender.

Nutrition

Per Serving: 310 calories; protein 19.7g; carbohydrates 57.9g; fat 1g; sodium 255.1mg.

Eggplant Dip

Prep:

20 mins

Cook:

22 mins

Additional:

10 mins

Total:

52 mins

Servings:

12

Yield:

2 cups

Ingredients

1 (8 ounce) can tomato sauce
¼ cup red wine vinegar
1 teaspoon salt
1 teaspoon white sugar
¼ teaspoon ground cayenne
2 tablespoons olive oil
1 tablespoon ground cumin
2 cloves garlic, minced
1 red bell pepper, seeded and cut into chunks
½ cup chopped fresh cilantro
1 ½ pounds eggplant, unpeeled, cut into chunks

Directions

1

Mix tomato sauce, red wine vinegar, cumin, salt, sugar, and cayenne together in a small bowl.

2

Heat olive oil in a large skillet over medium-low heat. Add garlic; cook and stir until golden, about 2 minutes. Add eggplant and red bell pepper; pour in tomato sauce mixture. Simmer, covered, until eggplant and red bell pepper soften, about 20 minutes. Remove from heat and let cool, about 10 minutes.

3

Transfer eggplant mixture to a food processor; pulse until it reaches the desired consistency. Sprinkle cilantro over dip.

Nutrition

Per Serving: 47 calories; protein 1.1g; carbohydrates 6g; fat 2.6g; sodium 295mg.

Red Pepper Tapenade

Prep:

20 mins

Total:

20 mins

Servings:

8

Yield:

8 appetizer servings

Ingredients

1 cup sun-dried tomatoes, packed in oil, drained and oil reserved

⅓ cup reserved sun-dried tomato oil

2 teaspoons balsamic vinegar

5 cloves garlic, finely chopped

6 ounces crumbled feta cheese

2 tablespoons dried basil

3 tablespoons finely chopped red pepper

½ teaspoon ground black pepper

Directions

1

Finely chop sun-dried tomatoes and place in a large bowl. Stir in the reserved tomato oil, red pepper, garlic, feta cheese, dried basil, black pepper, and balsamic vinegar and mix well. Cover and chill for at least four hours before serving.

Nutrition
Per Serving: 173 calories; protein 4.1g; carbohydrates 5.5g; fat 15.6g; cholesterol 18.9mg; sodium 275mg.

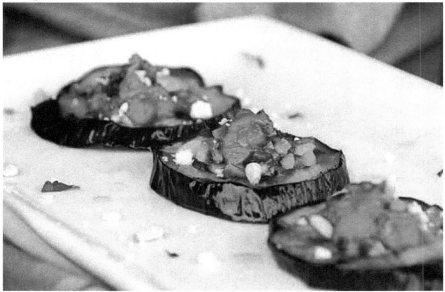

Halibut Pan

Prep:

15 mins

Cook:

10 mins

Total:

25 mins

Servings:

4

Yield:

4 servings

Ingredients

1 egg
1 cup all-purpose flour
2 tablespoons olive oil
1 teaspoon seafood seasoning (such as Old Bay®)
ground black pepper
1 pound skinless, boneless halibut fillets
1 teaspoon salt
2 tablespoons dried herbes de Provence

Directions

1

Whisk egg in a small bowl.

2

Combine flour, herbes de Provence, seafood seasoning, salt, and black pepper in a separate small bowl.

3

Cut halibut into 4 equal pieces.

4

Heat olive oil in a large frying pan over medium-low heat.

5

Dip each piece of halibut in whisked egg.

6

Dredge all sides of each piece in flour mixture to evenly coat; tap off excess flour.

7

Place coated pieces immediately in the hot olive oil.

8

Cook the halibut until lightly browned, about 5 minutes; turn and cook until fish is opaque and flakes easily with a fork, another 2 minutes.

Nutrition

Per Serving: 323 calories; protein 29.1g; carbohydrates 25.5g; fat 10.5g; cholesterol 83.1mg; sodium 787mg.

Fish and Tomato Sauce

Servings:
8

Yield:
8 servings

Ingredients

3 ½ ounces sun-dried tomatoes
½ cup grated Parmesan cheese
2 tablespoons olive oil
1 large yellow onion, chopped
2 (8 ounce) bottles clam juice
2 (14 ounce) cans diced tomatoes (no salt added)
1 cup dry red wine (or substitute broth or tomato juice)
4 garlic cloves, crushed
1 green bell pepper, chopped
4 tablespoons fresh herbs (such as thyme, rosemary or basil)
2 bay leaves
½ cup kalamata olives, sliced
1 pound firm fish (grouper, tilapia or tuna), cut in 2- to 3-inch chunks
2 teaspoons fennel seeds, lightly crushed
1 (15 ounce) can navy beans, drained and rinsed
1 pinch Salt and pepper, to taste

Directions
1

In a pan, simmer sun-dried tomatoes in 1 1/2 cups water until very soft; discard water.

2

In a large pot, saute onion and green pepper in oil until softened.

3

In a food processor or blender, combine sun-dried tomatoes and 1 bottle clam juice until smooth; add to pot. Stir in remaining clam juice, diced tomatoes, wine, garlic, herbs, bay leaves and olives. Simmer 20 minutes.

4

Add beans, fish, fennel seeds, salt and pepper. Simmer until fish is done, about 10 minutes. Remove bay leaves. Ladle into bowls; sprinkle with cheese.

Nutrition

Per Serving: 280 calories; protein 20.3g; carbohydrates 26g; fat 8.4g; cholesterol 26.5mg; sodium 839.9mg.

Pesto Dip

Prep:

15 mins

Total:

15 mins

Servings:

16

Yield:

2 cups

Ingredients

¼ cup chopped toasted walnuts
1 (8 ounce) package cream cheese, softened
2 tablespoons grated Parmesan cheese
6 tablespoons pesto
⅓ cup sour cream

Directions

1

In a medium bowl, blend cream cheese, sour cream and Parmesan cheese.

2

In a small clear glass serving dish, spread 1/3 the cream cheese mixture. Top with 2 tablespoons pesto. Repeat layering, ending with a topping of pesto. Sprinkle with walnuts and serve.

Nutrition

Per Serving: 103 calories; protein 2.8g; carbohydrates 1.2g; fat 9.9g; cholesterol 19.9mg; sodium 98.2mg.

Stuffed Zucchinis

Prep:

30 mins

Cook:

50 mins

Total:

1 hr 20 mins

Servings:

4

Yield:

4 servings

Ingredients

2 medium zucchini

½ pound mild sausage (such as Odom's Tennessee Pride® Mild Country Sausage)

½ tablespoon chopped fresh parsley

⅓ pound hot sausage (such as Odom's Tennessee Pride® Hot Country Sausage)

1 tablespoon butter

3 mushrooms, finely diced, or more to taste

¼ small onion, diced

½ stalk celery, diced

1 slice gluten-free bread, crumbled

1 tablespoon water

1 clove garlic, minced

⅛ cup grated Parmesan cheese

4 slices pepper Jack cheese

Directions

1

Preheat the oven to 375 degrees F.

2

Cut zucchini in half and scoop out and reserve interiors. Place zucchini halves close together in a casserole dish. Finely chop zucchini flesh and set aside in a bowl.

3

Heat a saucepan over medium-high heat. Add mild and hot sausage and cook until browned and crumbly, about 6 minutes. Drain and discard grease.

4

Melt butter in a frying pan over medium heat. Add chopped zucchini flesh, onion, mushrooms, celery, and garlic; cook and stir for 5 minutes. Stir in cooked sausage, bread crumbs, and enough water to hold the mixture together.

5

Spoon sausage mixture into zucchini boats, overflowing into the casserole dish.

6

Bake in the preheated oven for 30 minutes.

7

Remove from the oven, leaving oven on. Top with diced tomatoes, Parmesan cheese, and pepper Jack cheese, in that order. Return to the oven and cook until cheese is melted, about 10 minutes more. Top with parsley.

Nutrition

Per Serving: 488 calories; protein 21.3g; carbohydrates 10.3g; fat 38.7g; cholesterol 109.4mg; sodium 903.2mg.

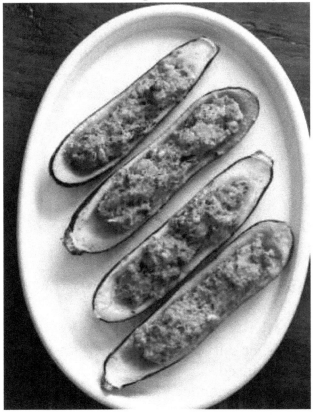

Creamy Chicken Curry

Prep:

20 mins

Cook:

30 mins

Additional:

4 hrs

Total:

4 hrs 50 mins

Servings:

8

Yield:

8 servings

Ingredients

For the Spice Mix:
2 teaspoons kosher salt
4 garlic cloves, minced
1 teaspoon ground coriander
2 teaspoons paprika
½ teaspoon cayenne pepper
1 ½ teaspoons ground cumin
½ teaspoon ground turmeric
2 teaspoons garam masala
1 tablespoon vegetable oil
2 tablespoons butter, divided
1 yellow onion, chopped
2 pounds boneless, skinless chicken thighs
2 tablespoons tomato paste
1 tablespoon minced fresh ginger root

1 cup chicken broth

2 cups cold water

¾ cup whole roasted cashews

⅓ cup freshly chopped cilantro

1 lime, juiced

⅓ cup sliced green onions

Directions

1

Mix salt, cumin, coriander, paprika, cayenne, turmeric, and garam masala together in a small bowl.

2

Cut a chicken thigh in half lengthwise along the crease. Halve the thicker portion to end up with three 2-inch pieces. Repeat with remaining chicken thighs.

3

Transfer chicken to a bowl. Add oil and about 1/2 of the spice blend; mix thoroughly. Cover with plastic wrap and marinate in the fridge for 4 to 12 hours.

4

Heat 1 tablespoon butter in a large pan over high heat until melted and golden brown. Add the chicken in a single layer. Cook until browned, 4 to 5 minutes per side. Return chicken and accumulated juices to the bowl.

5

Heat remaining butter in the same pan over medium-high heat. Add onion, remaining spice blend, tomato paste, garlic, and ginger. Cook and stir until fragrant, 2 to 3 minutes. Pour in chicken broth and bring to a simmer. Add the chicken and any accumulated juices.

6

Combine water and cashews in a blender; blend on high speed until very smooth. Stir cashew cream into the pan. Reduce heat to medium and simmer until flavors blend, 15 to 20 minutes. Stir in green onions and cilantro; taste for seasoning. Squeeze in lime juice.

Nutrition

Per Serving: 287 calories; protein 22g; carbohydrates 9.4g; fat 18.5g; cholesterol 76.8mg; sodium 823.9mg.

Fried Calamari

Prep:

15 mins

Cook:

10 mins

Total:

25 mins

Servings:

8

Yield:

8 servings

Ingredients

1 pound calamari tubes, thawed if frozen

peanut oil for frying

1 wedge lemon

6 cups all-purpose flour

4 eggs

1 tablespoon paprika

1 teaspoon salt

2 cups whole milk

1 teaspoon finely ground black pepper

1 tablespoon fresh parsley

Directions

1

Check calamari for breaks and slice into 1/8- to 1/4-inch rings.

2

Heat oil in a deep-fryer or large saucepan to 400 degrees F.

3

Place 2 cups flour in a bowl. Whisk milk and eggs together in a separate bowl. Place remaining 4 cups flour, cornstarch, paprika, salt, pepper, and cayenne in a third bowl; mix thoroughly.

4

Toss calamari rings in the plain flour. Move to the egg mixture and thoroughly coat. Move to the seasoned flour and coat fully. Move back to egg mixture if not thoroughly coated; coat with seasoned flour again.

5

Submerge floured calamari in the hot oil until golden, 3 to 4 minutes per batch. Lift out with a slotted spoon, letting oil drip off. Drain on paper towels. Place calamari in a small bowl; check seasoning. Add parsley and lemon wedge for garnish.

Nutrition

Per Serving: 523 calories; protein 22.9g; carbohydrates 79.8g; fat 11.6g; cholesterol 214.1mg; sodium 488.2mg.

Calamari Salad

Prep:

20 mins

Cook:

5 mins

Total:

25 mins

Servings:

12

Yield:

12 servings

Ingredients

2 lemons, juiced
4 stalks celery, chopped
6 cloves garlic, peeled and minced
salt and pepper to taste
3 pounds squid, cleaned and sliced into rounds
1 (2.25 ounce) can pitted black olives
1 sprig fresh parsley, chopped

Directions

1

In a medium bowl, mix lemon juice, garlic, and parsley.
Season with salt and pepper.

2

Bring a medium pot of water to a boil. Stir in squid, and cook
about 3 minutes, or until tender; drain.

3

Toss squid, olives, and celery with the lemon juice mixture. Cover, and chill in the refrigerator until serving.

Nutrition

Per Serving: 119 calories; protein 18.2g; carbohydrates 6.8g; fat 2.2g; cholesterol 264.5mg; sodium 108.5mg.

Wrapped Scallops

Prep:

15 mins

Cook:

10 mins

Total:

25 mins

Servings:

5

Yield:

10 appetizers

Ingredients

10 slices bacon

10 sea scallops

1 tablespoon olive oil

1 lemon, cut into wedges

1 teaspoon Cajun seasoning

Directions

1

Arrange bacon in a large skillet and cook over medium-high heat, turning occasionally, until lightly browned but still pliable, about 5 minutes. Drain the bacon slices on paper towels.

2

Wrap each slice of bacon around one sea scallop and secure with a toothpick. Season with Cajun seasoning.

3

Heat olive oil in a clean skillet over medium-high heat; sear scallops until golden and bacon is crisp, 3 to 4 minutes on each side. Squeeze lemon over scallops. Serve immediately.

Nutrition

Per Serving: 198 calories; protein 21.1g; carbohydrates 3.1g; fat 10.9g; cholesterol 54.4mg; sodium 683mg

Rainbow Chili

Prep:

20 mins

Cook:

1 hr 15 mins

Total:

1 hr 35 mins

Servings:

8

Yield:

8 servings

Ingredients

2 tablespoons olive oil

1 zucchini, sliced

1 (15 ounce) can black beans, drained and rinsed

1 yellow squash, sliced

1 red bell pepper, diced

¼ teaspoon cayenne pepper

1 green bell pepper, diced

4 cloves garlic, minced

1 onion, chopped

1 (28 ounce) can crushed tomatoes, with liquid

1 fresh jalapeno pepper, diced

1 (6 ounce) can tomato paste

1 (15 ounce) can whole kernel corn, drained

1 (15 ounce) can chili beans in spicy sauce, undrained

1 tablespoon chili powder

½ teaspoon dried oregano

½ teaspoon ground black pepper

Directions

1

Heat oil in a large pot over medium-high heat. Stir in zucchini, yellow squash, red bell pepper, green bell pepper, jalapeno, garlic, and onion. Cook 5-6 minutes, just until tender.

2

Mix tomatoes with liquid, tomato paste, black beans, corn, and chili beans in spicy sauce into the pot. Season with chili powder, oregano, black pepper, and cayenne pepper. Bring to a boil. Reduce heat to low and simmer 1 hour, stirring occasionally.

Nutrition

Per Serving: 188 calories; protein 7.4g; carbohydrates 33.8g; fat 5g; sodium 670.2mg.

Chicken Kebabs

Prep:

25 mins

Cook:

35 mins

Total:

1 hr

Servings:

4

Yield:

4 servings

Ingredients

4 tablespoons mild harissa paste or sauce

2 tablespoons honey

4 boneless, skinless chicken breasts, cut into 1-inch cubes

2 yellow squash, thickly sliced

2 green zucchini, thickly sliced

½ lemon, juiced

1 red onion, thickly sliced

2 cups thickly sliced button mushrooms

1 tablespoon ground cumin

½ teaspoon salt and pepper

3 tablespoons olive oil

Reynolds Wrap® Aluminum Foil

Directions

1

Preheat the oven to 425 degrees F.

2

Whisk together the harissa, honey and lemon juice in a bowl. Add chicken and mix until coated.

3

Skewer the chicken evenly among 8 wooden skewers and set aside.

4

Mix together the squash, zucchini, onion, mushrooms, olive oil, cumin and salt and pepper until completely combined.

5

Place a 1 1/2 to 2 feet long sheet of Reynolds Wrap® Aluminum Foil on a table and place 1/4 of the vegetables in the center of the foil. Place 2 chicken skewers on top of the vegetables. Fold up the ends and then the outside of the foil to create a foil packet.

6

Repeat the process 3 more times and place the foil packets on a cookie sheet.

7

Bake in the oven at 425 degrees F for 18-20 minutes and then open the foil packets and cook for a further 15 minutes or until the chicken is lightly browned and cooked throughout.

8

Optional Serving: Serve the individual foil packets alongside warm pita.

Nutrition

Per Serving: 321 calories; protein 27.9g; carbohydrates 23.1g; fat 14.3g; cholesterol 64.6mg; sodium 445.7mg.

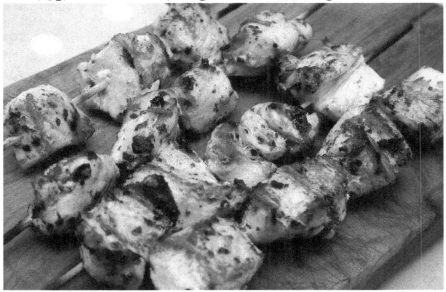

Chicken Wings

Prep:

5 mins

Cook:

1 hr

Total:

1 hr 5 mins

Servings:

6

Yield:

12 wings

Ingredients

12 large chicken wings, tips removed and wings cut in half at joint

1 cup water

1 tablespoon minced garlic

½ cup white sugar

⅓ cup soy sauce

1 tablespoon honey

2 teaspoons wine vinegar

2 tablespoons peanut butter

Directions

1

In an electric skillet or a large skillet over medium heat, mix together the water, sugar, soy sauce, peanut butter, honey, wine vinegar, and garlic until smooth and the sugar has dissolved. Place the wings into the sauce, cover, and simmer for 30 minutes. Uncover and simmer until the wings are tender and the sauce has thickened, about 25-30 more minutes, spooning sauce over wings occasionally. Sprinkle with sesame seeds.

Nutrition

Per Serving: 529 calories; protein 36.2g; carbohydrates 22.4g; fat 32.4g; cholesterol 141.7mg; sodium 962.5mg.

Salsa Verde

Prep:

15 mins

Total:

15 mins

Servings:

8

Yield:

8 servings

Ingredients

⅔ cup roasted, salted almonds, finely chopped
1 clove garlic, minced
1 bunch flat-leaf parsley, finely chopped
1 cup olive oil

Directions

1

Combine chopped almonds and parsley on a cutting board; chop together again until very finely chopped.

2

Transfer almond mixture to a bowl and add garlic. Stir olive oil into almond mixture until a thick sauce forms.

Nutrition

Per Serving: 311 calories; protein 2.8g; carbohydrates 2.8g; fat 33.1g; sodium 43.8mg.

Cinnamon Duck Mix

Prep:
10 mins

Cook:
10 mins

Total:
20 mins

Servings:
24

Yield:
12 cups

Ingredients

5 cups honey graham cereal

2 cups ramen noodles, crushed

¾ cup sliced almonds

3 cups cinnamon-flavored bear-shaped graham cookies

1 cup golden raisins

⅓ cup honey

1 teaspoon orange juice

⅓ cup butter

Directions

1

Preheat oven to 375 degrees F.

2

In a large bowl, mix honey graham cereal, bear-shaped graham cookies, ramen noodles, almonds, and golden raisins.

3

In a small saucepan over low heat, melt butter, and blend in honey and orange juice. Spread over the honey graham cereal mixture, and toss to coat.

4

Spread mixture onto a large baking sheet. Bake 10 minutes in the preheated oven.

Nutrition

Per Serving: 161 calories; protein 2g; carbohydrates 25.4g; fat 6.3g; cholesterol 6.8mg; sodium 213.3mg.

Ginger Duck

Prep:

10 mins

Cook:

30 mins

Total:

40 mins

Servings:

2

Yield:

2 servings

Ingredients

2 duck breast halves

1 teaspoon lime juice

1 pinch chili powder

1 pinch salt

1 pinch cayenne pepper

1 pinch ground black pepper

2 tablespoons honey

2 tablespoons soy sauce

2 tablespoons rice wine

1 tablespoon grated fresh ginger

½ cup chicken stock

1 tablespoon tomato sauce

Directions

1

Preheat oven to 400 degrees F.

2

Use a sharp knife to score across the duck breasts 4 times through the skin and fat but just barely to the meat. Rub the skin with salt, cayenne, and black pepper.

3

Preheat an ovenproof skillet over medium-high heat. Lay the breasts in the skillet skin-side down and fry until the skin is brown and crisp, about 5 minutes. Use a spoon to carefully discard any excess fat from the bottom of the skillet. Turn the breasts over and cook for 1-2 minute.

4

Place the skillet into the preheated oven and roast until the internal temperature of the thickest part of the breasts reach 160 degrees F for well done, or the breasts reach desired doneness.

5

Remove the duck breasts from the skillet and cover with foil. Set aside to rest. Pour off excess fat from the skillet. Place the stock, honey, soy sauce, rice wine, ginger, tomato sauce, chili powder, and lime juice in the skillet. Whisk the sauce over high heat, bring to a boil and cook until the sauce thickens, about 2 minutes. Slice the duck breasts thinly, arrange on serving plates, and pour the sauce over the top.

Nutrition

Per Serving: 260 calories; protein 20.6g; carbohydrates 21.3g; fat 8.8g; cholesterol 106mg; sodium 1186mg.

Duck Sauce

Prep:

20 mins

Cook:

40 mins

Additional:

30 mins

Total:

1 hr 30 mins

Servings:

8

Yield:

8 Cups

Ingredients

5 cups coarsely chopped mixed fruit (apples, plums, and pears)

½ teaspoon dry mustard

1 cup water

1 teaspoon soy sauce

1 tablespoon apricot preserves

½ cup packed light brown sugar

½ teaspoon garlic powder

¾ cup apple juice

Directions

1

Place fruit in a stock pot over medium high heat. Add water, apple juice, soy sauce, apricot preserves, brown sugar, garlic powder, and dry mustard. Bring to a simmer, stirring frequently to dissolve brown sugar. Reduce heat, and continue simmering for 40 minutes, or until fruit is completely soft. Remove from heat and allow to cool.

2

Blend sauce in a food processor or blender until completely smooth, adjusting consistency with additional water, if desired. Cover, and refrigerate until ready to use.

Nutrition

Per Serving: 224 calories; protein 2.4g; carbohydrates 55.9g; fat 0.4g; sodium 47.6mg.

Cucumber and Mango Salad

Prep:

20 mins

Total:

20 mins

Servings:

4

Yield:

4 servings

Ingredients

1 pound cucumbers, ends trimmed

1 ½ pounds mangos - peeled, pitted, and cut into 1-inch cubes

2 teaspoons sesame seeds

1 teaspoon agave nectar

½ teaspoon rice vinegar

Directions

1

Peel the cucumber in wide stripes lengthwise, alternating skinned strips with peel. Slice into 1/4-inch pieces and place into salad bowl.

2

Add mangos, rice vinegar, sesame seeds, and agave nectar to bowl and toss to blend.

Nutrition

Per Serving: 141 calories; protein 1.9g; carbohydrates 34.8g; fat 1.3g; sodium 5.8mg.

Chicken and Mint Sauce

Prep:

10 mins

Total:

10 mins

Servings:

6

Yield:

6 servings

Ingredients

1 teaspoon salt

freshly ground black pepper to taste

2 plum tomatoes, chopped

2 teaspoons Dijon mustard

½ teaspoon white suga

⅔ cup extra-virgin olive oil

¼ cup white wine vinegar

⅓ cup chopped fresh mint

Directions

1

Whisk together the olive oil, vinegar, salt, pepper, Dijon mustard, and sugar in a large bowl. Stir in the mint and tomatoes.

Nutrition

Per Serving: 237 calories; protein 0.5g; carbohydrates 2.8g; fat 25g; sodium 432.9mg.

Chewy Chestnuts

Prep:
15 mins

Cook:
20 mins

Additional:
12 hrs

Total:
12 hrs 35 mins

Servings:
4

Yield:
4 servings

Ingredients

1 (8 ounce) can water chestnuts, drained
1 (18 ounce) bottle barbeque sauce
½ pound sliced bacon

Directions

1

Wrap water chestnuts with bacon, securing with toothpicks. Arrange on a large baking sheet. Cover with barbecue sauce. Marinate in the refrigerator 12 to 24 hours.

2

Preheat oven to 300 degrees F.

3

Remove wrapped water chestnuts from the marinade and place on another large baking sheet. Bake 20 minutes in the preheated oven, or until the bacon is evenly brown but not too crisp.

Nutrition

Per Serving: 477 calories; protein 7.1g; carbohydrates 52.9g; fat 26g; cholesterol 38.6mg; sodium 1887.1mg.

Cumin Pork

Prep:
10 mins
Cook:
15 mins
Total:
25 mins
Servings:
2
Yield:
2 servings

Ingredients

½ teaspoon salt
ground black pepper to taste
1 tablespoon ground cumin
2 tablespoons olive oil, divided
1 tablespoon ground coriander
3 cloves garlic, minced
2 boneless pork loin chops

Directions
1
Mix the salt, cumin, coriander, garlic, and 1 tablespoon olive oil to form a paste. Season the pork chops with salt and pepper, and rub with the paste.

2

Heat the remaining olive oil in a skillet over medium heat, and cook the pork chops about 5 minutes on each side, to an internal temperature of 145 degrees F.

Nutrition
Per Serving: 278 calories; protein 15.5g; carbohydrates 4.8g; fat 22g; cholesterol 38.2mg; sodium 615.3mg.

Oregano Feta

Servings:

16

Yield:

1 cup

Ingredients

1 ¼ cups crumbled feta cheese
4 ounces cream cheese
Ground black pepper
1 teaspoon dried oregano

Directions

1

Place 1 cup feta in the work bowl of a food processor; process until fine-textured. Add cream cheese, oregano and pepper; process until smooth. Scrape into a bowl; stir in remaining feta. Transfer to a serving bowl or storage container.

Nutrition

Per Serving: 56 calories; protein 2.2g; carbohydrates 0.8g; fat 5g; cholesterol 18.2mg; sodium 151.8mg.

Orange Lamb and Potatoes

Prep:

30 mins

Cook:

1 hr

Total:

1 hr 30 mins

Servings:

4

Yield:

4 servings

Ingredients

1 large orange, juiced

1 (3 pound) half leg of lamb, bone-in

3 tablespoons dark French mustard

4 teaspoons dried oregano

salt and pepper to taste

3 tablespoons olive oil

10 potatoes, peeled and cut into 2-inch pieces

5 cloves garlic

Directions

1

Preheat oven to 375 degrees F.

2

In large bowl, whisk together the orange juice, mustard, olive oil, oregano, salt, and pepper. Stir the potatoes into the bowl to coat with orange juice mixture. Remove potatoes with a slotted spoon, and place them into a large roasting pan.

3

Cut slits into the lamb meat, and stuff the garlic cloves into the slits. Rub remaining orange juice mixture from bowl all over the lamb, and place the lamb on top of the potatoes in the roasting pan. If there's any remaining orange juice mixture, pour it over the lamb.

4

Roast in the preheated oven until the potatoes are tender and the lamb is cooked to medium, about 1 hour. A meat thermometer inserted into the thickest part of the meat should read 140 degrees F. Check every 20 to 30 minutes while roasting, and add a bit of hot water if you find the potatoes are drying out. If the lamb finishes cooking before the potatoes, remove the lamb to a cutting board or serving platter and cover with foil while the potatoes continue to bake in the oven.

Nutrition

Per Serving: 912 calories; protein 51.4g; carbohydrates 103.2g; fat 32.5g; cholesterol 137.1mg; sodium 311.6mg.

Lamb Ribs

Prep:

10 mins

Cook:

1 hr 10 mins

Additional:

1 hr

Total:

2 hrs 20 mins

Servings:

6

Yield:

6 servings

Ingredients

3 ½ pounds lamb ribs

1 teaspoon ground black pepper

2 onions, chopped

1 cup dry white wine

¼ cup soy sauce

¼ cup fresh lemon juice

1 tablespoon honey

1 tablespoon olive oil

2 teaspoons minced garlic

1 teaspoon ground cinnamon

1 teaspoon salt

Directions

1

Place lamb in a 9x13-inch baking dish.

2

Combine onions, white wine, soy sauce, lemon juice, honey, olive oil, garlic, cinnamon, salt, and pepper in a small bowl. Mix well and pour mixture all over lamb. Cover with plastic wrap and marinate in the refrigerator for 1 hour.

3

Preheat oven to 400 degrees F.

4

Roast lamb in the preheated oven until browned and tender, about 1 hour 10 minutes.

Nutrition

Per Serving: 508 calories; protein 25.8g; carbohydrates 10.2g; fat 36.8g; cholesterol 112.2mg; sodium 1077.1mg.

Lamb and Raisins

Prep:

15 mins

Cook:

1 hr 20 mins

Total:

1 hr 35 mins

Servings:

6

Yield:

6 servings

Ingredients

¼ cup butter

1 tablespoon olive oil

1 tablespoon ground cumin

6 (4 ounce) lamb chops

3 cups chopped onion

1 clove garlic, crushed

2 tablespoons curry powder

1 tablespoon ground coriander

2 teaspoons salt

2 teaspoons white pepper1 teaspoon dried thyme

½ lemon (including peel), seeded and finely chopped

3 cups apples - peeled, cored, and chopped

1 cup applesauce

1 teaspoon dried thyme

⅔ cup dark raisins

⅔ cup golden raisins

1 teaspoon seasoned salt

Directions

1

In a saucepan over medium heat, melt the butter with olive oil, and cook the onions and garlic until the onion is translucent, about 8 minutes. Stir in curry powder, coriander, cumin, salt, white pepper, thyme, lemon, apples, applesauce, dark raisins, and golden raisins until thoroughly combined. Bring the mixture to a boil, turn down the heat to a simmer, cover, and simmer the sauce until it has the consistency of applesauce and the raisins are plump and starting to break apart, about 1 hour. Mix in a tablespoon of water if sauce starts to become too thick.

2

Preheat an outdoor grill for medium heat, and lightly oil the grate. Sprinkle the lamb chops with seasoned salt.

3

Grill on the preheated grate until the chops are well-browned, cooked to your desired color of pink inside, and show grill marks, 3 to 5 minutes per side for medium-rare. An instant-read thermometer inserted into the center of a chop, not touching bone, should read about 145 degrees C. Serve the lamb chops with the sauce on the side.

Nutrition

Per Serving: 500 calories; protein 20g; carbohydrates 50.5g; fat 26.6g; cholesterol 87.5mg; sodium 1046.3mg.

Turmeric Pork and Mushrooms

Prep:

15 mins

Cook:

25 mins

Total:

40 mins

Servings:

4

Yield:

4 servings

Ingredients

1 tablespoon olive oil

4 bone-in pork chops

1 (10.75 ounce) can golden mushroom soup (such as Campbell's®)

1 teaspoon ground black pepper

1 tablespoon olive oil

1 (6 ounce) package sliced fresh mushrooms

1 teaspoon garlic salt

2 tablespoons water

Directions

1

Heat 1 tablespoon olive oil in a large skillet over medium heat. Sprinkle pork chops with garlic salt and black pepper. Fry pork chops in the hot oil until browned, 6 to 8 minutes per side. Transfer chops to a plate.

2

Heat 1 tablespoon olive oil in skillet; cook and stir mushrooms in the hot oil until soft, about 7 minutes. Scrape up and dissolve any browned bits of food into mushrooms as you stir. Pour golden mushroom soup and water into skillet and stir into mushrooms.

3

Place pork chops and accumulated juices into mushroom sauce, spooning sauce over chops. Simmer until meat is no longer pink inside and juices run clear, occasionally spooning more sauce over chops as they cook, 10 to 13 minutes.

Nutrition

Per Serving: 367 calories; protein 29g; carbohydrates 8g; fat 23.9g; cholesterol 75.1mg; sodium 1035.5mg.

Allspice Cheese Cream Mix

Prep:

20 mins

Total:

20 mins

Servings:

10

Yield:

3 cups

Ingredients

⅓ cup butter, softened

¾ teaspoon ground allspice

1 teaspoon vanilla extract

2 tablespoons milk

1 (3 ounce) package cream cheese, softened

4 cups confectioners' sugar

Directions

1

In a medium bowl, blend the cream cheese, butter, and allspice. Gradually mix in the confectioners' sugar, vanilla, and milk until the mixture is spreadable.

Nutrition

Per Serving: 274 calories; protein 0.8g; carbohydrates 48.3g; fat 9.2g; cholesterol 25.9mg; sodium 70.6mg

Leeks Salad

Prep:

10 mins

Additional:

2 hrs

Total:

2 hrs 10 mins

Servings:

20

Yield:

2.5 cups

Ingredients

¾ cup chopped leeks

salt and pepper to taste

1 (8 ounce) package cream cheese, softened

1 tablespoon white sugar

½ (12 ounce) jar bacon bits

1 cup creamy salad dressing

1 tablespoon white vinegar

Directions

1

In a medium bowl, mix together the leeks, cream cheese, creamy salad dressing, vinegar, sugar, bacon bits, salt and pepper. Refrigerate 2 to 3 hours, until well chilled.

Nutrition

Per Serving: 110 calories; protein 4.5g; carbohydrates 3g; fat 8.9g; cholesterol 22.3mg; sodium 397.8mg.

Zucchini and Corn

Prep:

20 mins

Cook:

20 mins

Additional:

5 mins

Total:

45 mins

Servings:

8

Yield:

8 servings

Ingredients

2 tablespoons vegetable oil

6 medium zucchini, sliced

½ pound shredded Monterey Jack cheese

½ medium onion, chopped

1 (14.5 ounce) can diced tomatoes, drained

2 teaspoons garlic powder

salt and pepper to taste

½ pound shredded sharp Cheddar cheese

1 (15.25 ounce) can whole kernel corn, drained

Directions

1

Heat oil in a medium saucepan over medium heat, and saute the zucchini and onion 6 to 7 minutes, until onion is tender. Mix in the corn. Stir in the diced tomatoes. Season with garlic powder, salt, and pepper. Cover, and cook 15 minutes, or until zucchini is soft.

2

Remove the saucepan from heat. Mix in the Monterey Jack cheese and Cheddar cheese. Cover, and let stand until cheeses are melted, about 5 minutes.

Nutrition

Per Serving: 333 calories; protein 17.8g; carbohydrates 18.3g; fat 22.2g; cholesterol 55mg; sodium 582.2mg.

Lime Salad

Servings:

8

Yield:

8 servings

Ingredients

1 (6 ounce) package lime flavored Jell-O® mix
1 cup shredded cabbage
¾ cup boiling water
½ cup grated carrots
¼ teaspoon salt
¾ cup cold water
½ cup chopped walnuts

Directions

1

Dissolve gelatin mix in boiling water. Stir in salt. Stir in cold water. Chill until slightly thickened.

2

Fold cabbage, carrots, and nuts into thickened gelatin. Pour mixture into an 8 inch mold that has been sprayed with a non-stick spray. Chill until firm.

3

Set mold in a sink of hot water for a few seconds when ready to unmold. Place serving plate on top of mold, and turn over. Lift off mold.

Nutrition

Per Serving: 129 calories; protein 3.2g; carbohydrates 20.3g; fat 4.8g; sodium 174.6mg.

Tomato and Feta Salad

Prep:

10 mins

Total:

10 mins

Servings:

4

Yield:

4 servings

Ingredients

4 teaspoons white wine vinegar

2 tablespoons chopped fresh basil

4 teaspoons olive oil

1 pint cherry tomatoes, halved

2 tablespoons finely chopped shallot

¼ cup crumbled feta cheese

¼ teaspoon coarse salt

Directions

1

Whisk vinegar, olive oil, and salt in a salad bowl. Stir in cherry tomatoes, shallot, feta cheese, and basil.

Nutrition

Per Serving: 103 calories; protein 3g; carbohydrates 5g; fat 8.4g; cholesterol 14mg; sodium 329.1mg.

Lettuce and Onions Salad

Prep:

10 mins

Cook:

10 mins

Total:

20 mins

Servings:

4

Yield:

4 servings

Ingredients

4 slices bacon

1 head leaf lettuce - rinsed, dried and torn into bite-size pieces

4 green onions, chopped

Directions

1

Place the bacon in a large, deep skillet, and cook over medium-high heat, turning occasionally, until evenly browned and crisp, about 10 minutes. Place the bacon slices on a paper towel-lined plate.

2

Add the chopped green onions to the bacon grease; cook and stir for about a minute or until the onions reach your desired tenderness. Pour the onions and bacon grease over the lettuce and toss lightly. Crumble the bacon and add it to the lettuce. Serve immediately.

Nutrition

Per Serving: 144 calories; protein 4.5g; carbohydrates 3.2g; fat 12.7g; cholesterol 19mg; sodium 255.2mg.

Carrot Salad

Prep:

15 mins

Total:

15 mins

Servings:

8

Yield:

8 servings

Ingredients

4 carrots, shredded

¼ cup blanched slivered almonds

1 apple - peeled, cored and shredded

2 tablespoons honey

1 tablespoon lemon juice

salt and pepper to taste

Directions

1

In a bowl, combine the carrots, apple, lemon juice, honey, almonds, salt and pepper. Toss and chill before serving.

Nutrition

Per Serving: 58 calories; protein 1.1g; carbohydrates 10.5g; fat 1.8g; sodium 21.8mg

CHAPTER 4: SNACK RECIPES

Zucchini Chips

Prep:

10 mins

Cook:

2 hrs

Total:

2 hrs 10 mins

Servings:

2

Yield:

2 servings

Ingredients

2 large large zucchini, thinly sliced
1 tablespoon olive oil, or to taste
sea salt to taste

Directions

1

Preheat oven to 250 degrees F.

2

Arrange sliced zucchini on a baking sheet. Drizzle lightly with olive oil and sprinkle lightly with sea salt.

3

Bake in the preheated oven until completely dried and chip-like, about 1 hour per side. Allow to cool before serving.

Nutrition

Per Serving: 111 calories; protein 3.9g; carbohydrates 10.8g; fat 7.3g; sodium 192.4mg.

Hummus Snack Bowl

Prep:

10 mins

Total:

10 mins

Servings:

8

Yield:

8 servings

Ingredients

2 (15 ounce) cans garbanzo beans, drained and liquid reserved

6 tablespoons olive oil

3 cloves garlic

1 teaspoon salt

5 tablespoons lemon juice

1 teaspoon ground coriander

⅛ teaspoon cayenne pepper

⅛ teaspoon ground cumin

Directions

1

Combine garbanzo beans, olive oil, lemon juice, garlic, salt, coriander, cumin, and cayenne in a food processor. Add 4 tablespoons reserved bean liquid and process until hummus is smooth.

Nutrition

Per Serving: 177 calories; protein 3.6g; carbohydrates 16.6g; fat 11g; sodium 500.5mg.

Roasted Almonds

Prep:

5 mins

Cook:

1 hr

Additional:

25 mins

Total:

1 hr 30 mins

Servings:

12

Yield:

3 cups almonds

Ingredients

1 egg white
¼ teaspoon salt
1 teaspoon vanilla extract
3 cups whole almonds
½ cup brown sugar
1 teaspoon ground cinnamon
½ cup white sugar
1 teaspoon chili powder

Directions

1

Preheat oven to 250 degrees F. Lightly grease a 10x15-inch jelly roll pan.

2

Combine egg white and vanilla in large bowl; beat until frothy. Add almonds and toss to coat. Pour almonds into a mesh strainer to drain excess liquid, 5 to 10 minutes. Return strained almonds to the bowl.

3

Stir white sugar, brown sugar, cinnamon, chili powder, and salt together in a bowl. Sprinkle sugar mixture over almonds and toss to coat evenly. Spread coated nuts evenly onto prepared jelly roll pan.

4

Bake, stirring every 20 minutes, until the seasoning clings to the almonds, about 1 hour. Allow to cool completely before storing in an air-tight container.

Nutrition
Per Serving: 276 calories; protein 7.9g; carbohydrates 24.7g; fat 18g; sodium 58.3mg.

Feta Fettuccini

Prep:

10 mins

Cook:

10 mins

Total:

20 mins

Servings:

6

Yield:

6 servings

Ingredients

1 pound fresh fettuccine pasta
2 tablespoons extra virgin olive oil
5 ripe tomatoes, chopped
½ small red onion, chopped
½ cup pitted kalamata olives, chopped
freshly ground black pepper to taste
1 cup chopped fresh basil
1 cup crumbled feta cheese

Directions

1

Bring a large pot of lightly salted water to a boil. Add fettuccini and cook for 7 to 10 minutes or until al dente; drain.

2

In a medium bowl combine tomatoes, onion, basil, olives and black pepper.

3

Toss the fettuccini with olive oil. Serve pasta topped with tomato mixture and feta cheese.

Nutrition

Per Serving: 494 calories; protein 16.1g; carbohydrates 71.3g; fat 17.3g; cholesterol 22.3mg; sodium 933.2mg.

Hummus Dip

Prep:

10 mins

Total:

10 mins

Servings:

8

Yield:

8 servings

Ingredients

1 (15 ounce) can chickpeas, drained

½ teaspoon curry powder

2 (6 ounce) jars artichoke hearts, drained

½ cup Greek yogurt

½ cup fresh basil

¼ cup olive oil

1 lemon, juiced

⅓ cup pickled jalapeno pepper slices

2 tablespoons hemp seeds

2 cloves garlic

1 teaspoon ground cayenne pepper

1 teaspoon ground paprika

Directions

1

Combine chickpeas, artichoke hearts, Greek yogurt, basil, jalapeno pepper slices, olive oil, lemon juice, hemp seeds, garlic, paprika, cayenne pepper, and curry powder in a food processor; blend until smooth.

Nutrition

Per Serving: 160 calories; protein 5.1g; carbohydrates 14.5g; fat 9.6g; cholesterol 2.8mg; sodium 410.7mg.

Crispy Seedy Crackers

Prep:

20 mins

Cook:

12 mins

Total:

32 mins

Servings:

60

Yield:

5 dozen crackers

Ingredients

1 ½ cups all-purpose flour
½ cup cold water
1 ½ teaspoons kosher salt
½ cup freshly grated Parmigiano-Reggiano cheese
1 teaspoon white sugar
3 tablespoons extra-virgin olive oil
1 tablespoon minced fresh rosemary

Directions

1

Preheat oven to 400 degrees F. Line a baking sheet with a silicon mat or parchment paper.

2

Place flour, salt, sugar, and grated cheese in a mixing bowl. Stir together until well mixed. Add rosemary; drizzle with olive oil and add water. Mix with a fork until mixture comes together in a fairly sticky dough and pulls away from the sides of the bowl, 3 to 5 minutes.

3

Transfer dough onto floured surface and add flour as you knead the dough. Knead until it no longer sticks to work surface, 4 to 5 minutes. Divide dough in half.

4

Dust work surface with flour. Roll out dough to 1/8-inch thickness or less. Brush or mist surface of dough very lightly with water. Sprinkle with coarse sea salt. Prick the entire surface of dough with the tines of a fork to prevent crackers from puffing too much when baking.

5

Cut each rolled out half into about 30 pieces with a pizza wheel. You can cut them out in squares, rectangles, or triangles--your choice. Transfer onto prepared baking sheet with a bench scraper or your floured fingers (dough will be very sticky).

6

Bake in preheated oven until perfectly browned and crunchy, 10 to 15 minutes, depending on the thickness.

Nutrition

Per Serving: 21 calories; protein 0.6g; carbohydrates 2.5g; fat 0.9g; cholesterol 0.6mg; sodium 58.3mg.

Cucumber Boats

Prep:

10 mins

Total:

10 mins

Servings:

4

Yield:

4 servings

Ingredients

1 (5 ounce) can chunk light tuna in water, drained

2 cucumbers, halved lengthwise and seeded

¼ cup chopped carrot

3 tablespoons low-fat plain Greek-style yogurt

2 tablespoons diced red onion

1 tablespoon mayonnaise

¼ cup chopped celery

¼ cup chopped broccoli

Directions

1

Mix tuna, carrot, celery, broccoli, yogurt, red onion, and mayonnaise together in a bowl; spread into the cucumber halves.

Nutrition

Per Serving: 96 calories; protein 10.2g; carbohydrates 7.5g; fat 3.2g; cholesterol 10.8mg; sodium 55.6mg.

Beef Paprika

Prep:

10 mins

Cook:

2 hrs 30 mins

Total:

2 hrs 40 mins

Servings:

7

Yield:

6 to 8 servings

Ingredients

2 pounds lean beef chuck, trimmed and cut into 1 inch cubes

1 cup chopped onion

2 tablespoons all-purpose flour

1 clove garlic, minced

¾ cup ketchup

2 tablespoons Worcestershire sauce

¼ cup shortening

2 teaspoons salt

½ teaspoon mustard powder

2 teaspoons paprika

1 tablespoon brown sugar

1 ½ cups water

¼ cup water

Directions

1

Melt shortening in large skillet over medium high heat. Add meat, onion, and garlic; cook and stir until meat is browned.

2

Stir in ketchup, Worcestershire sauce, brown sugar, salt, paprika, mustard and 1 1/2 cup water. Reduce heat, cover, and simmer 2 to 2 1/2 hours.

3

Blend flour and 1/4 cup water. Stir into meat. Heat to boiling, stirring constantly. Serve hot.

Nutrition
Per Serving: 426 calories; protein 23.5g; carbohydrates 13.7g; fat 30.8g; cholesterol 92mg; sodium 1088.4mg.

Baked Dark Chocolate Lava Cake

Prep:

15 mins

Cook:

15 mins

Additional:

5 mins

Total:

35 mins

Servings:

6

Yield:

6 cakes

Ingredients

8 ounces 70% bittersweet chocolate, finely chopped

½ cup granulated sugar

⅛ teaspoon salt

12 tablespoons cold unsalted butter, cut into cubes

4 large eggs

Directions

1

Preheat oven to 375 degrees F. Adjust a rack to the middle of the oven. Butter six 4-ounce ramekins.

2

Put the chocolate and butter in a metal or glass bowl over barely simmering water. Stir occasionally until melted. Remove from the heat.

3

Place the eggs, sugar, and salt in the bowl of a mixer. Whip at medium-high speed until light and fluffy, about 5 minutes. Reduce speed to low and add the chocolate; mix until combined. Spoon into the prepared ramekins and place on a baking sheet.

4

Bake for about 10 minutes or until the edges are set but the center is underdone. Let cool 3 minutes before serving.

Nutrition

Per Serving: 525 calories; protein 7g; carbohydrates 38.3g; fat 38.9g; cholesterol 186.7mg; sodium 100.1mg.

Air Fried Popcorn Shrimp

Prep:

15 mins

Cook:

20 mins

Additional:

5 mins

Total:

40 mins

Servings:

4

Yield:

4 servings

Ingredients

12 ounces large shrimp, peeled and deveined
1 cup panko bread crumbs
¼ cup all-purpose flour
1 egg
⅛ teaspoon ground black pepper
½ teaspoon paprika
½ teaspoon onion powder
¼ teaspoon salt
nonstick cooking spray

Directions

1

Place shrimp in a large bowl. Sprinkle flour over the top and toss until shrimp are evenly coated in flour. Beat egg in a separate bowl. Combine panko bread crumbs, paprika, onion powder, salt, and pepper in a third bowl.

2

Dip each flour-coated shrimp in egg, toss in panko mixture, and place on a baking sheet. Let rest for 5 minutes while the air fryer is preheating.

3

Preheat air fryer to 400 degrees F for 5-6 minutes.

4

Spray the basket of the air fryer with cooking spray. Arrange 1/2 of the shrimp in the basket. Mist the top of each shrimp with cooking spray.

5

Cook for 4 minutes. Using tongs, flip each shrimp over and mist any chalky spots with cooking spray. Cook 4 minutes more. Repeat with remaining shrimp.

Nutrition

Per Serving: 182 calories; protein 19g; carbohydrates 25.2g; fat 2.9g; cholesterol 174.2mg; sodium 442.9mg.

Spicy Shrimp

Prep:

15 mins

Cook:

20 mins

Total:

35 mins

Servings:

4

Yield:

1 pound

Ingredients

2 tablespoons vegetable oil

2 onions, chopped

1 pound peeled and deveined shrimp

1 tomato, chopped

1 teaspoon garlic paste

2 green chile peppers, seeded and minced

salt to taste

½ teaspoon ground turmeric

½ teaspoon garam masala

¼ cup cilantro leaves

Directions

1

Heat oil over medium-high heat in a large skillet, and cook and stir onions until golden brown, about 8 minutes. Stir in tomato and cook for 2 minutes. Stir in garlic paste, turmeric, garam masala, green chile peppers, and salt, and cook for 2 minutes more.

2

Reduce heat to low, add the shrimp, and cook and stir over low heat until the shrimp are bright pink on the outside and the meat is no longer transparent in the center, about 8 minutes. Add a small amount of water if needed; the sauce should be thick. Sprinkle with cilantro.

Nutrition

Per Serving: 215 calories; protein 20.6g; carbohydrates 14.6g; fat 8.2g; cholesterol 172.6mg; sodium 250.9mg.

Honey Walnuts

Prep:

5 mins

Cook:

10 mins

Total:

15 mins

Servings:

6

Yield:

6 servings

Ingredients

10 walnut halves

¼ cup orange blossom honey

1 (8 ounce) package cream cheese (such as Philadelphia®), softened

Directions

1

Preheat oven to 350 degrees F.

2

Place walnuts on a baking sheet. Bake until toasted and fragrant, about 10 minutes. Transfer walnuts to a plate to cool. When walnuts are cool, transfer to a resealable plastic bag and crush with a rolling pin.

3

Combine cream cheese, honey, and walnuts in a food processor and pulse until creamy.

Nutrition

Per Serving: 195 calories; protein 3.4g; carbohydrates 13.1g; fat 15.2g; cholesterol 41.1mg; sodium 111.1mg.

Bacon-Wrapped Dates Stuffed with Manchego Cheese

Prep:

10 mins

Cook:

10 mins

Total:

20 mins

Servings:

8

Yield:

24 dates

Ingredients

4 ounces manchego cheese, cut into 24 small cubes

24 dried pitted dates

24 wooden toothpicks

8 slices bacon, cut into thirds

Directions

1

Preheat oven to 400 degrees F.

2

Stuff 1 piece manchego cheese into each date and then wrap with 1 piece bacon, securing with a toothpick. Arrange dates in a shallow baking dish with the bacon seam down and 1 inch between pieces.

3

Bake in preheated oven for 5 minutes, turn dates with tongs, and continue baking until bacon is crisp, 5 to 7 minutes more. Drain on a plate lined with paper towels.

Nutrition

Per Serving: 167 calories; protein 6.7g; carbohydrates 19.5g; fat 7.3g; cholesterol 20.2mg; sodium 407.4mg.

Orange Baked Olives

Prep:

25 mins

Cook:

15 mins

Total:

40 mins

Servings:

12

Yield:

3 cups

Ingredients

3 ½ cups whole mixed olives, drained

¼ cup dry white wine

4 teaspoons grated orange zest

2 tablespoons fresh orange juice

2 cloves garlic, minced

2 sprigs fresh rosemary

2 tablespoons fresh parsley, chopped

1 ½ tablespoons chopped fresh oregano

¼ teaspoon crushed red pepper flakes

2 tablespoons olive oil

Directions

1

Preheat oven to 375 degrees F. Stir the olives together with
the wine, orange juice, olive oil, and garlic in a 9x13 inch
baking dish. Nestle the sprigs of rosemary in the olives.

2

Bake in the preheated oven for 15 minutes, stirring halfway through the baking. Remove and discard the rosemary sprigs, then stir in the parsley, oregano, orange zest, and red pepper flakes. Serve warm, or cool the olives and use them to top a salad.

Nutrition

Per Serving: 75 calories; protein 0.7g; carbohydrates 1.4g; fat 7.5g; sodium 980.9mg.

Spicy Roasted Potatoes

Prep:

15 mins

Cook:

40 mins

Total:

55 mins

Servings:

4

Yield:

4 servings

Ingredients

5 medium red potatoes, diced with peel

1 tablespoon garlic powder

1 tablespoon kosher salt

2 teaspoons chili powder

¼ cup extra virgin olive oil

1 medium onion, chopped

Directions

1

Preheat the oven to 450 degrees F.

2

Arrange the potatoes and onions in a greased 9x13 inch baking dish so that they are evenly distributed. Season with garlic powder, salt and chili powder. Drizzle with olive oil. Stir to coat potatoes and onions with oil and spices.

3

Bake for 35 to 40 minutes in the preheated oven, until potatoes are fork tender and slightly crispy. Stir every 10 minutes. When done, sprinkle with cheese. Wait about 5 minutes for the cheese to melt before serving.

Nutrition

Per Serving: 473 calories; protein 14.4g; carbohydrates 47.6g; fat 26.1g; cholesterol 36.2mg; sodium 1685.1mg.

Pecan Almond Bars

Prep:

15 mins

Cook:

35 mins

Additional:

30 mins

Total:

1 hr 20 mins

Servings:

18

Yield:

18 servings

Ingredients

1 cup almonds

2 tablespoons all-purpose flour

¼ teaspoon salt

⅛ teaspoon baking powder

⅛ teaspoon baking soda

1 cup pecan halves

2 tablespoons flax seeds

¼ cup quick-cooking oats

5 tablespoons maple syrup

1 teaspoon vanilla extract

1 cup pitted and quartered dates

Directions

1

Preheat oven to 350 degrees F.

2

Spread pecans and almonds onto a baking sheet.

3

Bake in the preheated oven until nuts are toasted and fragrant, 7 to 8 minutes. Remove baking sheet from oven and decrease oven temperature to 325 degrees F.

4

Combine flour, flax seeds, salt, baking powder, and baking soda in a food processor; pulse a few times. Add pecans and almonds to flour mixture; pulse until nuts are coarsely chopped. Add oats and dates to flour-nut mixture; pulse just until combined.

5

Whisk maple syrup and vanilla extract together in a bowl until smooth; pour over oat mixture and pulse just until combined. Spread oat mixture into an 8-inch square pan.

6

Bake in the preheated oven lightly browned, about 25 minutes; cool to room temperature.

Nutrition

Per Serving: 140 calories; protein 2.9g; carbohydrates 14.1g; fat 9g; sodium 45.7mg.

Air Fried Sweet Potato Chips

Prep:

10 mins

Cook:

10 mins

Total:

20 mins

Servings:

2

Yield:

2 servings

Ingredients

1 sweet potatoes, peeled and cut into 1/2 inch wide fries

¼ teaspoon pepper

1 tablespoon canola oil

⅛ teaspoon ground sweet paprika

½ teaspoon kosher salt

⅛ teaspoon garlic powder

Directions

1

Preheat the air fryer to 400 degrees F.

2

Combine sweet potato fries and canola oil in a bowl and mix. Season with salt, pepper, garlic powder, and paprika. Mix until all fries are evenly coated.

3

Divide sweet potatoes into 2 or 3 batches for cooking. Place an even layer of sweet potatoes in the fry basket, insert in the air fryer, and cook until golden, about 10 minutes. Repeat with remaining sweet potatoes.

Nutrition
Per Serving: 119 calories; protein 1.1g; carbohydrates 13.5g; fat 7.1g; sodium 516mg.

CHAPTER 5: DESSERTS

Muhalabieh

Prep:
10 mins
Cook:
15 mins
Additional:
2 hrs
Total:
2 hrs 25 mins
Servings:
6
Yield:
6 servings

Ingredients

3 cups milk
2 cardamom pods, crushed
¾ cup white sugar
6 tablespoons cornstarch
1 cup heavy whipping cream
1 tablespoon rose water
1 cup cold water

Directions

1

Combine milk and sugar together in a saucepan; bring to a boil.

2

Whisk water and cornstarch together in a bowl until smooth; stir into boiling milk. Cook milk mixture over medium heat until thickened to the consistency of cake batter, 15 to 20 minutes. Remove saucepan from heat and stir cream, rose water, and cardamom into milk mixture.

3

Refrigerate milk mixture until completely cooled, 2 to 4 hours.

Nutrition

Per Serving: 326 calories; protein 4.9g; carbohydrates 39.3g; fat 17.1g; cholesterol 64.1mg; sodium 67mg.

Panna Cotta

Prep:

10 mins

Cook:

10 mins

Additional:

4 hrs 15 mins

Total:

4 hrs 35 mins

Servings:

6

Yield:

6 servings

Ingredients

2 tablespoons freshly squeezed lemon juice

3 cups heavy cream

½ cup white sugar

2 ½ tablespoons fresh lemon zest, divided

1 (.25 ounce) package powdered gelatin (such as Knox®)

Directions

1

Place lemon juice in a small bowl and sprinkle the unflavored gelatin over it. Let stand for about 15 minutes until gelatin softens.

2

Combine heavy cream, sugar, and 2 tablespoons lemon zest in a saucepan over medium-low heat; bring to a simmer. Whisk in gelatin mixture until dissolved. Remove from heat and stir in orange liqueur.

3
Strain the cream mixture into a medium bowl and divide evenly among small glass bowls or ramekins.

4
Place uncovered panna cottas into the refrigerator until set, at least 4 hours. If time permits, cover the bowls with plastic wrap and chill overnight.

5
Garnish with remaining lemon zest before serving.

Nutrition
Per Serving: 488 calories; protein 3.5g; carbohydrates 21.4g; fat 44g; cholesterol 163mg; sodium 47.8mg.

Cherry Cream

Prep:

20 mins

Additional:

30 mins

Total:

50 mins

Servings:

8

Yield:

8 servings

Ingredients

1 (12 ounce) can cherry pie filling

1 (3 ounce) package cream cheese, softened

¼ teaspoon almond extract

½ cup confectioners' sugar

1 cup heavy whipping cream

½ teaspoon vanilla extract

1 (9 inch) pie shell, baked

Directions

1

In a small bowl, combine cream cheese, confectioners' sugar, vanilla, and almond extracts. Beat with an electric mixer until light and fluffy. In a separate medium bowl, beat whipping cream until stiff. Carefully fold cream cheese mixture into whipped cream.

2

Spread beaten mixture in the bottom of pie crust. Cover with cherry pie filling. Refrigerate pie until set and cold, about 30 minutes.

Nutrition

Per Serving: 338 calories; protein 3g; carbohydrates 31.4g; fat 22.5g; cholesterol 52.4mg; sodium 172.4mg.

Strawberries Cream

Prep:

15 mins

Cook:

30 mins

Total:

45 mins

Servings:

12

Yield:

12 servings

Ingredients

½ cup butter, melted
1 cup milk
½ teaspoon salt
2 cups fresh strawberry halves
1 cup all-purpose flour
1 cup white sugar
2 teaspoons baking powder
1 (4 ounce) package cream cheese, cut into small pieces

Directions

1
Preheat oven to 400 degrees F.

2
Pour melted butter into the bottom of a 9x13-inch glass baking dish.

3

Mix milk, flour, sugar, baking powder, and salt together in a small bowl; pour over the butter in the baking dish. Arrange strawberry halves in a layer into the baking dish. Dot the strawberries with the cream cheese pieces.

4

Bake in preheated oven until top is golden brown and edges are bubbling, 30 to 40 minutes.

Nutrition

Per Serving: 222 calories; protein 2.7g; carbohydrates 28g; fat 11.5g; cholesterol 32.3mg; sodium 269.3mg.

Anise Cookies

Prep:

15 mins

Cook:

15 mins

Additional:

1 hr

Total:

1 hr 30 mins

Servings:

40

Yield:

40 servings

Ingredients

Cookies:
4 large eggs
1 teaspoon anise oil
1 cup white sugar
¾ cup vegetable oil
2 tablespoons baking powder
5 cups all-purpose flour
Icing:
½ cup confectioners' sugar
2 tablespoons milk

Directions

1

Beat eggs together in a large bowl. Gradually stir white sugar into beaten eggs until smooth. Slowly pour vegetable oil and anise oil into sugar mixture until incorporated. Mix flour and baking powder together in a separate bowl; slowly add to sugar mixture, stirring with a wooden spoon until dough is dry.

2

Refrigerate dough, 30 minutes to overnight.

3

Preheat oven to 350 degrees F. Lightly grease a baking sheet.

4

Roll dough into walnut-size balls and arrange on the prepared baking sheet.

5

Bake in the preheated oven until cookies are crisp around the edges, 12 to 15 minutes. Cool cookies on baking sheet for 5 minutes before transferring to a wire rack.

6

Mix confectioners' sugar and milk together in a bowl until desired consistency is reached. Dip a fork into the icing and drizzle over cookies. Allow icing to harden.

Nutrition

Per Serving: 128 calories; protein 2.3g; carbohydrates 18.7g; fat 4.9g; cholesterol 18.7mg; sodium 80.8mg.

Cocoa Brownies

Prep:

10 mins

Cook:

28 mins

Additional:

10 mins

Total:

48 mins

Servings:

12

Yield:

1 9x11-inch pan

Ingredients

2 cups hot cocoa mix
1 cup all-purpose white flour
¼ cup milk
¾ cup butter
2 cups white sugar
3 eggs
2 teaspoons vanilla extract

Directions

1

Preheat oven to 350 degrees F. Grease a 9x11-inch baking pan.

2

Place hot cocoa mix and butter in a large microwave-safe bowl; microwave until butter is mostly melted, about 3 minutes. Stir well. Add sugar, eggs, and vanilla extract and mix thoroughly. Add milk; mix until batter is thick and creamy. Mix in flour.

3

Bake in the preheated oven in 5 to 10 minute increments until set and sticky in texture, 25 to 65 minutes. Let cool for 10 minutes before cutting into bars.

Nutrition

Per Serving: 376 calories; protein 4.4g; carbohydrates 59.6g; fat 13.8g; cholesterol 77.4mg; sodium 209.1mg.

Plum Cake

Prep:
20 mins

Cook:
40 mins

Total:
1 hr

Servings:
8

Yield:
1 9-inch cake

Ingredients

3 eggs
1 cup all-purpose flour
½ cup butter, softened
½ cup white sugar
1 ¼ cups plums, pitted and quartered
1 teaspoon lemon zest
½ teaspoon baking powder

Directions

1

Preheat oven to 375 degrees F. Grease and flour one 9-inch tube pan.

2

Separate the eggs. In a small bowl, beat the egg whites until stiff peaks form, and set aside.

3

In a large bowl, cream the butter and sugar. Beat in the egg yolks and the lemon zest.

4

Stir together the flour and baking powder and then blend the flour mixture into the creamed mixture. Gently fold in the egg whites. Spread the batter evenly into the prepared pan. There will only be a little over an inch of batter. Arrange the plums, skin side down, attractively over the batter.

5

Bake in preheated oven until a tester inserted in the center comes out clean, about 40 minutes. Transfer to a cooling rack and allow to cool before serving.

Nutrition

Per Serving: 246 calories; protein 4.3g; carbohydrates 27.6g; fat 13.6g; cholesterol 100.3mg; sodium 138.8mg.

Sesame Cookies

Servings:

24

Yield:

4 dozen

Ingredients

½ cup butter

1 teaspoon vanilla extract

½ teaspoon baking powder

¾ cup confectioners' sugar

1 egg

1 ¼ cups all-purpose flour

¾ cup sesame seeds, toasted

¼ teaspoon salt

Directions

1

To Toast Sesame Seeds: Pour seeds into a pie pan and place in a 300 degrees F oven for about 10 minutes or until lightly browned. Stir seeds occasionally.

2

Cream the butter or margarine with the vanilla until light and fluffy. Add the confectioners' sugar gradually, beating until fluffy. Add egg and beat thoroughly.

3

Sift the flour, baking powder and salt together. Add in thirds to the creamed mixture. After each addition of the flour mixture stir in the toasted sesame seeds. Mix until blended. Cover and chill dough for at least 2 hours.

4

Preheat oven to 350 degrees F.

5

On a lightly floured surface, roll 1/3 of the dough at a time to 1/8 inch thick. Cut with a 2 inch scalloped cutter. Transfer cookies to ungreased cookie sheets.

6

Bake at 350 degrees F for 9 to 12 minutes.

Nutrition

Per Serving: 102 calories; protein 1.8g; carbohydrates 9.8g; fat 6.3g; cholesterol 17.9mg; sodium 65.2mg.

Catalan Cookies

Prep:

1 hr

Cook:

15 mins

Total:

1 hr 15 mins

Servings:

24

Yield:

24 cookies

Ingredients

1 pound small potatoes, scrubbed

1 egg white

1 cup almonds

1 cup chopped almonds

1 cup white sugar

Directions

1

Place potatoes in a saucepan with enough water to cover. Bring to a boil, and cook until tender, 20 to 30 minutes. When done, you can stab them with a fork, and they will fall off easily. Drain, cool slightly, and peel.

2

Preheat the oven to 350 degrees F.

3

Place 1 cup of almonds into a food processor, and grind to a fine powder. Add sugar to almonds, and process to mix. Transfer to a medium bowl. Add potatoes to the almond mixture, and mash together until it becomes a very thick paste. Roll into 1 inch balls, and roll the balls in chopped almonds. Place cookies on a baking sheet, and brush with egg white.

4

Bake for 10 to 15 minutes in the preheated oven, until the tops are brown. Gently remove from the baking sheets, and cool on a plate in the refrigerator. Serve cold. They are supposed to be squishy when you eat them.

Nutrition

Per Serving: 116 calories; protein 3g; carbohydrates 14g; fat 6g; sodium 3.6mg.

Lepinja

Prep:

30 mins

Cook:

20 mins

Additional:

2 hrs

Total:

2 hrs 50 mins

Servings:

12

Yield:

1 loaf

Ingredients

2 tablespoons warm milk (110 to 115 degrees F)
2 ⅓ cups all-purpose flour
1 teaspoon salt
1 tablespoon white sugar
1 (.25 ounce) package active dry yeast
1 cup warm water (110 to 115 degrees F)

Directions

1

Sprinkle the yeast over the warm milk in a small bowl. Let stand for 5 minutes until the yeast softens and begins to form a creamy foam. Stir the warm water and sugar into the yeast mixture.

2

Stir the flour and salt together in a separate bowl; add all but about 1/2 cup of the flour mixture to the yeast mixture; mix with your hands until a soft dough forms, adding the last of the flour mixture a little at a time until it clears the sides of the bowl. Cover the bowl with a light cloth and let the dough rise in a warm place (80 to 95 degrees F) until doubled in volume, about 1 hour.

3

Deflate, or 'punch down,' the dough and turn out onto a work surface lightly dusted with flour; knead for about 5 minutes. Return the dough to the bowl, cover again with a light cloth, and allow the dough to again rise until doubled in volume, about 30 minutes more.

4

Preheat an oven to 400 degrees F . Lightly grease a baking sheet.

5

Deflate the dough and turn turn out onto a work surface lightly dusted with flour; knead lightly. Place the dough onto the prepared baking sheet; shape into an oval about 1/2-inch thick. Set aside to rise a third time for about 30 minutes.

6

Bake in the preheated oven until nicely browned and hollow sounding when thumped, 20 to 25 minutes.

Nutrition

Per Serving: 96 calories; protein 2.8g; carbohydrates 19.9g; fat 0.3g; cholesterol 0.2mg; sodium 196.2mg

Sweet Rice Pudding

Prep:

5 mins

Cook:

40 mins

Total:

45 mins

Servings:

4

Yield:

4 servings

Ingredients

1 ½ cups water
½ cup long grain rice
1 cup 2% milk
½ cup white sugar
1 tablespoon butter
1 pinch ground cinnamon
½ (12 fluid ounce) can evaporated milk

Directions

1

Bring water and rice to a boil in a saucepan. Reduce heat to medium-low, cover, and simmer until rice is tender and water has been absorbed, about 20. Add 2% milk, evaporated milk, sugar, and butter; stir well and cook until creamy, about 20 minutes longer. Serve sprinkled with cinnamon.

Nutrition

Per Serving: 301 calories; protein 6.9g; carbohydrates 51.3g; fat 7.8g; cholesterol 26.2mg; sodium 99.4mg.

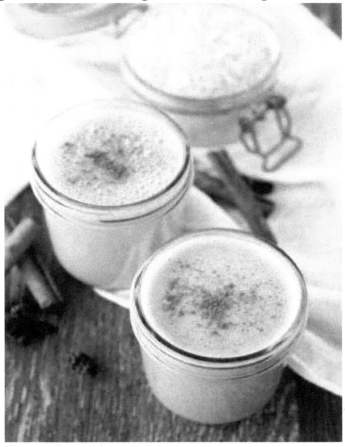

Fruit Crepes

Prep:

10 mins

Cook:

10 mins

Total:

20 mins

Servings:

4

Yield:

4 servings

Ingredients

4 (7 inch) pre-made crepes
1 cup chocolate hazelnut spread
1 (7 ounce) can pressurized whipped cream
4 bananas, sliced

Directions

1

Spread 1/4 cup of chocolate hazelnut spread onto each crepe.
Arrange 1 sliced banana down the center of each one. Roll up,
and place in a warm skillet over medium heat. Let them warm
up for about 90 seconds. Transfer to plates, and serve topped
with whipped cream.

Nutrition

Per Serving: 639 calories; protein 9.7g; carbohydrates 81.6g;
fat 32.9g; cholesterol 87.3mg; sodium 226.6mg.

Crème Caramel

Servings:

60

Yield:

4 to 5 dozen caramels

Ingredients

2 cups white sugar
1 pint heavy whipping cream
1 cup butter
1 cup corn syrup
1 cup evaporated milk
1 ¼ teaspoons vanilla extract
1 cup packed brown sugar

Directions

1

Grease a 12x15 inch pan.

2

In a medium-size pot, combine sugar, brown sugar, corn syrup, evaporated milk, whipping cream, and butter. Monitor the heat of the mixture with a candy thermometer while stirring. When the thermometer reaches 250 degrees F remove the pot from the heat.

3

Stir in vanilla. Transfer mixture to the prepared pan and let the mixture cool completely. When cooled cut the Carmel into small squares and wrap them in wax paper for storage.

Nutrition

Per Serving: 115 calories; protein 0.5g; carbohydrates 14.8g; fat 6.3g; cholesterol 20.2mg; sodium 30.4mg.

Ripe Banana Pudding

Prep:

10 mins

Cook:

10 mins

Total:

20 mins

Servings:

4

Yield:

2 cups

Ingredients

2 cups milk

½ cup ground oats

1 large banana, cut into 1/2-inch slices

⅓ cup white sugar

1 tablespoon cornstarch

⅓ cup raisins

1 tablespoon butter

1 egg

Directions

1

Whisk milk, oats, sugar, egg, and cornstarch together in a saucepan over medium heat; add banana and raisins. Cook, stirring constantly, until pudding is thick, 10 to 15 minutes. Remove from heat and stir in butter. Spoon pudding into dessert dishes.

Nutrition

Per Serving: 293 calories; protein 7.9g; carbohydrates 50.9g; fat 7.8g; cholesterol 63.9mg; sodium 90mg.

Cioccolata Calda

Prep:

5 mins

Cook:

15 mins

Total:

20 mins

Servings:

2

Yield:

2 servings

Ingredients

3 tablespoons cocoa powder

1 tablespoon cornstarch

1 ½ cups milk

2 tablespoons milk

1 ½ tablespoons white sugar

Directions

1

Mix the cocoa powder and sugar together in a small saucepan. Stir the 1 1/2 cups milk into the saucepan until the sugar has dissolved. Place over low heat; slowly bring the mixture to a low simmer.

2

Whisk 2 tablespoons of milk together with the cornstarch in a small cup; slowly whisk the cornstarch slurry into the cocoa mixture. Continue cooking, whisking continually, until the hot chocolate reaches a pudding-like thickness, 2 to 3 minutes.

Nutrition
Per Serving: 169 calories; protein 8.1g; carbohydrates 26.7g; fat 5g; cholesterol 15.9mg; sodium 83.3mg

Chocolate Pudding

Prep:

5 mins

Cook:

15 mins

Additional:

3 hrs

Total:

3 hrs 20 mins

Servings:

6

Yield:

6 servings

Ingredients

3 cups whole milk, divided

⅓ cup white sugar

1 cup semisweet chocolate chips

¼ cup cornstarch

Directions

1

Combine 1/2 cup milk and cornstarch in a small bowl. Whisk or stir with a fork until smooth and all lumps have been incorporated.

2

Combine remaining milk with sugar in a medium saucepan over low heat. Slowly whisk in the cornstarch mixture. Cook, whisking as needed to prevent lumps from forming, until mixture begins to thicken, 8 to 10 minutes. Add chocolate chips and salt. Continue stirring until chips are completely melted and pudding is smooth and thickened, about 7 minutes more.

3

Pour pudding into 1 large bowl or 6 individual bowls. Place plastic wrap directly on top of the pudding to prevent a skin from forming; smooth it gently against the surface. Refrigerate for at least 3 to 4 hours before serving.

Nutrition

Per Serving: 271 calories; protein 5.1g; carbohydrates 39.2g; fat 12.4g; cholesterol 12.2mg; sodium 78.2mg.

Vanilla Cake

Prep:

20 mins

Cook:

30 mins

Total:

50 mins

Servings:

12

Yield:

1 9x9-inch cake

Ingredients

1 cup white sugar

1 ½ cups all-purpose flour

2 eggs

1 teaspoon vanilla extract

1 teaspoon almond extract

3 tablespoons cornstarch

1 ¾ teaspoons baking powder

½ cup butter

½ teaspoon salt

¾ cup milk

Directions

1

Preheat the oven to 350 degrees F. Grease and flour a 9x9-inch pan.

2

Beat sugar and butter together in a medium bowl until creamy. Beat in eggs, 1 at a time; stir in vanilla extract and almond extract.

3

Combine flour, cornstarch, baking powder, and salt in another bowl. Add to the creamed mixture and mix well. Stir in milk until batter is smooth. Pour or spoon batter into the prepared pan.

4

Bake in the preheated oven until it springs back to the touch, 30 to 40 minutes.

Nutrition

Per Serving: 219 calories; protein 3.3g; carbohydrates 31.4g; fat 9g; cholesterol 52.6mg; sodium 240.9mg.

Ekmek Kataifi

Prep:

1 hr

Cook:

40 mins

Additional:

4 days

Total:

4 days

Servings:

12

Yield:

2 loaves

Ingredients

1 ½ cups bread flour, divided
2 cups warm water (110 degrees F)
5 teaspoons active dry yeast
1 teaspoon white sugar
6 cups bread flour
2 teaspoons salt
¾ cup water, divided

Directions

1

To make the starter: Place 1/2 cup flour and 1/4 cup water in a coverable bowl; stir well. Cover and let sit at room temperature overnight. The next day, add 1/2 cup flour and 1/4 cup water to the bowl. Cover and let sit at room temperature overnight. On the third day, add 1/2 cup flour and 1/4 cup water to the bowl. Cover and let sit at room temperature overnight.

2

To make the dough: In a large bowl, dissolve the yeast and sugar in the warm water. Let stand until creamy, about 10 minutes.

3

Break the starter into small pieces and add it to the yeast mixture. Stir in 4 cups of flour and the salt. Stir in the remaining flour, 1/2 cup at a time, beating well after each addition. When the dough has pulled together, turn it out onto a lightly floured surface and knead until smooth and elastic, about 8 minutes. Sprinkle a little flour over the dough and then cover it with a dry cloth. Let it raise until double in size.

4

Put the dough back onto a lightly floured work surface and punch out the air. Divide the dough in half and knead each piece for 2 to 3 minutes. Shape each piece into a tight oval loaf. Sprinkle two sheet pans with corn meal. Roll and stretch two loaf until they are 15x12 inch ovals. Dust the tops of the loaves with flour. Cover with a dry cloth and let raise in a warm place until doubled in size. Meanwhile, preheat oven to 425 degrees F.

5

Bake in preheated oven for 30 to 40 minutes. Mist with water 3 times in the first 15 minutes. Loaves are done when their bottoms sound hollow when tapped. Let cool on wire racks before serving.

Nutrition
Per Serving: 6 calories; protein 0.6g; carbohydrates 1g; fat 0.1g; sodium 390mg.

Brownie Pops

Prep:

30 mins

Cook:

38 mins

Additional:

1 hr 15 mins

Total:

2 hrs 23 mins

Servings:

36

Yield:

36 brownie pops

Ingredients

cooking spray

2 (18.3 ounce) packages fudge brownie mix (such as Duncan Hines®)

½ cup water

1 cup vegetable oil

4 eggs

Ganache:

6 ounces semisweet chocolate chips

1 (16 ounce) package confectioners' coating (such as Wilton® Candy Melts®)

½ cup heavy whipping cream

lollipop sticks

Directions

1

Preheat oven to 350 degrees F. Coat an 11x15-inch baking pan with cooking spray.

2

Empty brownie mix into a large bowl. Add vegetable oil, eggs, and water; stir with a wooden spoon until batter is well blended. Pour batter into the prepared baking pan.

3

Bake in the preheated oven until a toothpick inserted 1 inch from the edge of the pan comes out clean, 35 to 40 minutes. Let cool completely, about 30 minutes.

4

Combine chocolate chips and heavy cream in a microwave-safe bowl. Heat in the microwave in 30-second intervals, stirring after each interval, until melted and smooth. Cool, about 5 minutes.

5

Break brownies into pieces and place in a large bowl. Pour ganache evenly over brownie pieces; mix thoroughly.

6

Line a jelly roll pan with parchment paper. Press brownie mixture evenly into the pan. Freeze until firm, about 30 minutes.

7

Pour confectioners' coating into a microwave-safe bowl. Microwave at 50 percent power for 1 minute; stir thoroughly. Continue to microwave and stir at 30-second intervals until smooth and completely melted, 1 to 2 minutes more.

8

Roll brownie mixture into balls; insert a lollipop stick halfway into each. Dip balls one at a time into melted confectioners' coating to form a thin, even coating, letting the excess drip off. Stick into a styrofoam block; let stand until coating hardens, about 10 minutes.

Nutrition

Per Serving: 284 calories; protein 3.4g; carbohydrates 32.7g; fat 16.6g; cholesterol 28.6mg; sodium 132.6mg.

Galaktoboureko

Prep:

1 hr

Cook:

45 mins

Total:

1 hr 45 mins

Servings:

15

Yield:

15 servings

Ingredients

6 cups whole milk

1 cup semolina flour

3 ½ tablespoons cornstarch

1 cup white sugar

¼ teaspoon salt

12 sheets phyllo dough

6 eggs

½ cup white sugar

¾ cup butter, melted

1 cup water

1 cup white sugar

1 teaspoon vanilla extract

Directions

1

Pour milk into a large saucepan, and bring to a boil over medium heat. In a medium bowl, whisk together the semolina, cornstarch, 1 cup sugar and salt so there are no cornstarch clumps. When milk comes to a boil, gradually add the semolina mixture, stirring constantly with a wooden spoon. Cook, stirring constantly until the mixture thickens and comes to a full boil. Remove from heat, and set aside. Keep warm.

2

In a large bowl, beat eggs with an electric mixer at high speed. Add 1/2 cup of sugar, and whip until thick and pale, about 10 minutes. Stir in vanilla.

3

Fold the whipped eggs into the hot semolina mixture. Partially cover the pan, and set aside to cool.

4

Preheat the oven to 350 degrees F .

5

Butter a 9x13 inch baking dish, and layer 7 sheets of phyllo into the pan, brushing each one with butter as you lay it in. Pour the custard into the pan over the phyllo, and cover with the remaining 5 sheets of phyllo, brushing each sheet with butter as you lay it down.

6

Bake for 40 to 45 minutes in the preheated oven, until the top crust is crisp and the custard filling has set. In a small saucepan, stir together the remaining cup of sugar and water. Bring to a boil. When the Galaktoboureko comes out of the oven, spoon the hot sugar syrup over the top, particularly the edges. Cool completely before cutting and serving. Store in the refrigerator.

Nutrition
Per Serving: 391 calories; protein 8.3g; carbohydrates 55.7g; fat 15.4g; cholesterol 108.6mg; sodium 244.9mg.

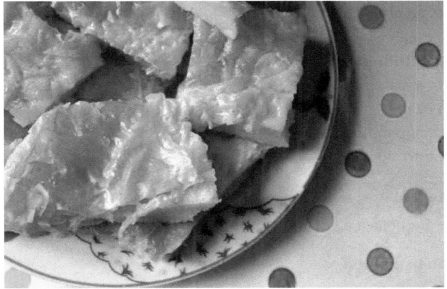

Ruby Cake

Prep:

30 mins

Cook:

45 mins

Additional:

15 mins

Total:

1 hr 30 mins

Servings:

12

Yield:

1 - 9x13 inch pan

Ingredients

CAKE:
2 cups all-purpose flour
1 ½ teaspoons baking soda
½ teaspoon salt
1 ½ cups white sugar
2 eggs
1 (15.25 ounce) can fruit cocktail with juice
TOPPING:
½ cup brown sugar
1 cup chopped walnuts
1 cup flaked coconut
SAUCE:
½ cup margarine
1 cup evaporated milk
1 cup flaked coconut

1 cup light corn syrup

Directions

1

Preheat oven to 350 degrees F. Grease and flour a 9x13 inch pan. Mix together the topping **Ingredients** - brown sugar, chopped nuts and 1 cup coconut. Set aside.

2

In a large bowl, mix together the flour, sugar, baking soda and salt. Make a well in the center and pour in the eggs and fruit cocktail with juice. Mix well and pour into prepared pan. Sprinkle with topping mixture.

3

Bake in the preheated oven for 30 to 35 minutes, or until a toothpick inserted into the center of the cake comes out clean.

4

In a saucepan, combine margarine, corn syrup, evaporated milk and flaked coconut. Cook, stirring constantly, until mixture boils and thickens. Pour over cake and place back in oven for few minutes until it bubbles.

Nutrition

Per Serving: 528 calories; protein 6.8g; carbohydrates 85.1g; fat 19.9g; cholesterol 37.1mg; sodium 432.5mg.

Pumpkin Cream

Prep:

15 mins

Total:

15 mins

Servings:

2

Yield:

2 coffees

Ingredients

½ cup heavy whipping cream

2 teaspoons pumpkin pie spice

3 tablespoons pumpkin pie syrup (such as Torani(R)), or to taste

ice

2 tablespoons sugar-free vanilla syrup (such as Torani®)

¼ cup pumpkin puree

1 cup cold brew coffee

Directions

1

Combine heavy whipping cream, pumpkin puree, pumpkin pie syrup, and pumpkin spice in a bowl. Whip with a hand mixer until creamy and slightly thickened.

2

Fill 2 glasses with ice. Add 1 tablespoon vanilla syrup to each glass, fill 2/3 of the way with cold brew coffee, and divide pumpkin cream evenly between both.

Nutrition

Per Serving: 223 calories; protein 1.8g; carbohydrates 5.3g; fat 22.3g; cholesterol 81.5mg; sodium 105.9mg.

Mandarin

Prep:

5 mins

Total:

5 mins

Servings:

1

Yield:

1 cocktail

Ingredients

1 fluid ounce mandarin vodka

1 twist lemon

2 fluid ounces syrup from a can of mandarin oranges

Directions

1

Pour the vodka and mandarin orange syrup into a cocktail shaker over ice. Cover, and shake until the outside of the shaker has frosted. Strain into a chilled martini glass, and garnish with a lemon twist to serve.

Nutrition

Per Serving: 86 calories; protein 0.4g; carbohydrates 5.8g; fat 0g; cholesterol 0mg; sodium 3.2mg.

Fruit Cobbler

Servings:
4
Yield:
4 servings

Ingredients

¾ cup all-purpose flour
¾ cup sugar
1 tablespoon sugar
1 teaspoon baking powder
¼ teaspoon salt
¾ cup milk
2 cups of sliced fresh peaches or nectarines, or whole
blueberries, strawberries, raspberries, blackberries or a
combination of fruits (or a 12-ounce package of frozen
berries)
4 tablespoons butter

Directions
1
Adjust oven rack to upper-middle position, and heat oven to
350 degrees.

2
Put butter in an 8-inch square or 9-inch round pan; set in
oven to melt. When butter has melted, remove pan from oven.

3

Whisk flour, 3/4 cup of sugar, baking powder and salt in small bowl. Add milk; whisk to form a smooth batter. Pour batter into pan, then scatter fruit over batter. Sprinkle with remaining 1 Tb. of sugar.

4

Bake until batter browns and fruit bubbles, 50 to 60 minutes. Serve warm or at room temperature with a dollop of whipped cream or a small scoop of vanilla ice cream, if desired.

Nutrition

Per Serving: 384 calories; protein 4.1g; carbohydrates 64.9g; fat 12.6g; cholesterol 34.2mg; sodium 370.8mg.

Black Forest

Servings:
18
Yield:
1 - 9 x 13 inch pan

Ingredients

1 (18.25 ounce) package devil's food cake mix with pudding
3 eggs
1 tablespoon butter
2 tablespoons milk
1 tablespoon almond extract
1 ½ cups semisweet chocolate chips
½ cup confectioners' sugar
1 (21 ounce) can cherry pie filling

Directions
1
Preheat oven to 350 degrees F.

2
Mix together: cake mix, beaten eggs, almond extract, cherry pie filling and 1 cup semisweet chocolate chips. Stir until just combined. Pour batter into a greased 9x13 inch pan.

3
Bake in a 350 degree F oven for 45 to 50 minutes or until a toothpick inserted in the center comes out clean. Remove cake from oven and let cool.

4

To Make Glaze: Heat 1/2 cup semisweet chocolate chips, butter or margarine, and milk in a saucepan over medium high heat. Once semisweet chocolate chips are melted and mixture is combined stir in confectioners' sugar.

5

Spread glaze over cooled cake. Serve cake as is or with whipped cream and a cherry.

Nutrition

Per Serving: 263 calories; protein 4.1g; carbohydrates 41.7g; fat 9.7g; cholesterol 38.5mg; sodium 235.7mg.

Tapioca Pudding

Prep:

10 mins

Cook:

15 mins

Total:

25 mins

Servings:

6

Yield:

6 servings

Ingredients

3 cups whole milk

¼ teaspoon salt

2 eggs, beaten

½ cup white sugar

½ teaspoon vanilla extract

½ cup quick-cooking tapioca

Directions

1

Stir together the milk, tapioca, sugar, and salt in a medium saucepan. Bring the mixture to a boil over medium heat, stirring constantly. Reduce heat to low; cook and stir 5 minutes longer.

2

Whisk 1 cup of the hot milk mixture into the beaten eggs, 2 tablespoons at a time until incorporated. Stir the egg mixture back into the tapioca until well mixed. Bring the pudding to a gentle simmer over medium-low heat; cook and stir 2 minutes longer until the pudding becomes thick enough to evenly coat the back of a metal spoon. Remove from the heat and stir in the vanilla. The pudding may be served hot or poured into serving dishes and refrigerated several hours until cold

Nutrition

Per Serving: 209 calories; protein 7.4g; carbohydrates 33g; fat 5.6g; cholesterol 74.2mg; sodium 169.1mg.

Banana Shake Bowls

Prep:

5 mins

Total:

5 mins

Servings:

1

Yield:

1 serving

Ingredients

1 (8 ounce) container Classic French Vanilla Flavor Ready-to-Drink CARNATION BREAKFAST ESSENTIALS® Complete Nutritional Drink
1 banana
4 ice cubes
1 tablespoon instant coffee crystals

Directions

1

Place all **Ingredients** in blender; cover. Blend until smooth. Pour into bowl and enjoy!

Nutrition

Per Serving: 351 calories; protein 11.6g; carbohydrates 69g; fat 4.4g; cholesterol 10mg; sodium 154.6mg.

Boozy Watermelon

Prep:

10 mins

Additional:

2 hrs

Total:

2 hrs 10 mins

Servings:

6

Yield:

6 servings

Ingredients

1 small watermelon, cut into 1-inch pieces

2 tablespoons turbinado sugar, or to taste

1 cup cachaca (Brazilian sugar cane spirit)

Directions

1

Place watermelon in a non-reactive container with a tight-fitting lid. Add cachaca and sugar. Cover container with the lid and shake until watermelon is coated and sugar is dissolved.

2

Refrigerate watermelon until watermelon is fully infused, 2 hours to overnight. Shake mixture again before serving.

Nutrition

Per Serving: 174 calories; protein 1.4g; carbohydrates 21.1g; fat 0.3g; sodium 4.3mg.

Chocolate Lava Cake

Prep:

15 mins

Cook:

15 mins

Additional:

5 mins

Total:

35 mins

Servings:

6

Yield:

6 cakes

Ingredients

12 tablespoons cold unsalted butter, cut into cubes

4 large eggs

⅛ teaspoon salt

½ cup granulated sugar

8 ounces 70% bittersweet chocolate, finely chopped

Directions

1

Preheat oven to 375 degrees F. Adjust a rack to the middle of the oven. Butter six 4-ounce ramekins.

2

Put the chocolate and butter in a metal or glass bowl over barely simmering water. Stir occasionally until melted. Remove from the heat.

3

Place the eggs, sugar, and salt in the bowl of a mixer. Whip at medium-high speed until light and fluffy, about 5 minutes. Reduce speed to low and add the chocolate; mix until combined. Spoon into the prepared ramekins and place on a baking sheet.

4

Bake for about 10 minutes or until the edges are set but the center is underdone. Let cool 3 minutes before serving.

Nutrition

Per Serving: 525 calories; protein 7g; carbohydrates 38.3g; fat 38.9g; cholesterol 186.7mg; sodium 100.1mg.

Lemon Squares

Prep:

25 mins

Cook:

25 mins

Additional:

2 hrs

Total:

2 hrs 50 mins

Servings:

16

Yield:

16 servings, one square each

Ingredients

20 Reduced Fat NILLA Wafers, finely crushed

½ cup flour

¼ cup firmly packed brown sugar

3 tablespoons grated lemon peel, divided

¼ cup fresh lemon juice

¼ cup cold margarine

1 cup granulated sugar

2 eggs

2 tablespoons flour

¼ teaspoon CALUMET Baking Powder

2 teaspoons powdered sugar

1 (8 ounce) package PHILADELPHIA Neufchatel Cheese, softened

Directions

1

Preheat oven to 350 degrees F. Line 8-inch square baking pan with foil, with ends of foil extending over sides of pan. Combine wafer crumbs, 1/2 cup flour and the brown sugar in bowl. Cut in margarine with pastry blender or two knives until mixture resembles coarse crumbs; press firmly onto bottom of prepared pan. Bake 15 min.

2

Meanwhile, beat Neufchatel cheese and granulated sugar with electric mixer on medium speed until well blended. Add eggs and 2 Tbsp. flour; mix well. Blend in 1 Tbsp. lemon peel, the lemon juice and baking powder; pour over crust.

3

Bake 25 to 28 min. or until center is set. Cool completely. Cover and refrigerate at least 2 hours or overnight. Sprinkle with powdered sugar and remaining 2 Tbsp. lemon peel just before serving.

Nutrition

Per Serving: 172 calories; protein 2.5g; carbohydrates 24.8g; fat 6.5g; cholesterol 33.3mg; sodium 128.4mg.

Ginger - Peach Jam

Prep:

10 mins

Cook:

25 mins

Total:

35 mins

Servings:

64

Yield:

8 cups

Ingredients

¼ cup finely chopped crystallized ginger

6 cups white sugar

½ teaspoon butter

4 ½ cups fresh peaches - peeled, pitted and chopped

1 (1.75 ounce) package powdered fruit pectin

Directions

1

Bring peaches, ginger, and pectin to a boil in a large saucepan over medium heat. Stir in the sugar and butter; cook and stir until the sugar is dissolved. Return to a boil, stirring constantly for 1 minute more. Remove from heat, and skim off any foam with a spoon.

2

Sterilize the jars and lids in boiling water for at least 5 minutes. Pack the peach jam into the hot, sterilized jars, filling the jars to within 1/4 inch of the top. Run a knife or a thin spatula around the insides of the jars after they have been filled to remove any air bubbles. Wipe the rims of the jars with a moist paper towel to remove any food residue. Top with lids, and screw on rings.

3

Place a rack in the bottom of a large stockpot and fill halfway with water. Bring to a boil over high heat, then carefully lower the jars into the pot using a holder. Leave a 2 inch space between the jars. Pour in more boiling water if necessary until the water level is at least 1 inch above the tops of the jars. Bring the water to a full boil, cover the pot, and process for 10 minutes.

4

Remove the jars from the stockpot and place onto a cloth-covered or wood surface, several inches apart, until cool. Once cool, press the top of each lid with a finger, ensuring that the seal is tight (lid does not move up or down at all). Store in a cool, dark area.

Nutrition
Per Serving: 76 calories; carbohydrates 19.6g; cholesterol 0.1mg; sodium 0.8mg.

Pear Jam

Prep:

20 mins

Cook:

15 mins

Additional:

1 hr

Total:

1 hr 35 mins

Servings:

64

Yield:

8 half-pint jars

Ingredients

4 ½ cups mashed ripe pears

¼ cup lemon juice

7 ½ cups white sugar

1 teaspoon ground cinnamon

½ teaspoon ground cloves

½ teaspoon ground allspice

½ teaspoon ground nutmeg

1 teaspoon butter

8 half-pint canning jars with lids and rings

3 tablespoons powdered fruit pectin

Directions

1

Mix pears, fruit pectin, cinnamon, cloves, allspice, nutmeg, and lemon juice in a large heavy pot; bring to a boil, stirring constantly. Add sugar all at once, stirring, and bring back to a full rolling boil. Boil for 1 minute. Mix in butter to settle foam.

2

Sterilize the jars and lids in boiling water for at least 5 minutes. Pack the pear jam into the hot, sterilized jars, filling the jars to within 1/4 inch of the top. Run a knife or a thin spatula around the insides of the jars after they have been filled to remove any air bubbles. Wipe the rims of the jars with a moist paper towel to remove any food residue. Top with lids, and screw on rings.

3

Place a rack in the bottom of a large stockpot and fill halfway with water. Bring to a boil and lower jars into the boiling water using a holder. Leave a 2-inch space between the jars. Pour in more boiling water if necessary to bring the water level to at least 1 inch above the tops of the jars. Bring the water to a rolling boil, cover the pot, and process for 10 minutes.

4

Remove the jars from the stockpot and place onto a cloth-covered or wood surface, several inches apart, until cool. Once cool, press the top of each lid with a finger, ensuring that the seal is tight (lid does not move up or down at all). Store in a cool, dark area.

Nutrition

Per Serving: 99 calories; protein 0.1g; carbohydrates 25.4g; fat 0.1g; cholesterol 0.2mg; sodium 0.6mg.

Grapefruit Marmalade

Prep:

20 mins

Cook:

35 mins

Additional:

1 day

Total:

1 day

Servings:

10

Yield:

2 5-ounce jars

Ingredients

4 ruby red grapefruits
3 cups white sugar

Directions

1

Inspect two 5-ounce jars for cracks and rings for rust, discarding any defective ones. Immerse in simmering water until marmalade is ready. Wash new, unused lids and rings in warm soapy water.

2

Thoroughly wash and dry the grapefruits. Run a zester around 2 grapefruits to produce ribbons of zest. Set aside. Cut away thin strips of peel from the other two grapefruits with a sharp paring knife.

3

Peel off all remaining outer white parts of the fruit and discard. Cut the grapefruits into wheels. Remove any seeds.

4

Put grapefruit wheels and zest strips into a non-reactive saucepan. Add sugar and stir well to cover fruit. Heat over medium-high heat until bubbling, mixing constantly. Smash the heated fruit until it liquefies. Reduce heat to low and cook over a steady boil, stirring often. Remove and discard any persistent white froth that won't disappear after being stirred. Continue to cook for about 10 minutes until marmalade begins to coat the back of a spoon.

5

Add zest ribbons and cook for 5 minutes more. Place a small amount of marmalade on a plate and put it in the freezer. Test the consistency after 3 minutes.

6

Remove the marmalade from the heat when the freezer sample meets your desired consistency.

7

Pack grapefruit jam into hot, sterilized jars, filling to within 1/4 inch of the top. Run a clean knife or thin spatula around the insides of the jars to remove any air bubbles. Wipe rims with a moist paper towel to remove any residue. Top with lids and screw rings on tightly.

8

Place a rack in the bottom of a large stockpot and fill halfway with water. Bring to a boil and lower jars 2 inches apart into the boiling water using a holder. Pour in more boiling water to cover jars by at least 1 inch. Bring to a rolling boil, cover, and process for 10 minutes.

9

Remove the jars from the stockpot and let rest, several inches apart, for 24 hours. Press the center of each lid with a finger to ensure the lid does not move up or down. Remove the rings for storage and store in a cool, dark area.

Nutrition
Per Serving: 276 calories; protein 0.8g; carbohydrates 71.1g; fat 0.1g.

Syrup Coffee

Prep:

10 mins

Total:

10 mins

Servings:

4

Yield:

4 cups

Ingredients

¼ cup instant coffee granules

1 (14 ounce) can sweetened condensed milk

2 cups hot water

Directions

1

Combine the instant coffee granules with the hot water and stir until dissolved. Stir in the condensed milk. Store in an airtight container or jar and refrigerate, until ready to use.

Nutrition

Per Serving: 321 calories; protein 8.1g; carbohydrates 54.3g; fat 8.5g; cholesterol 33.3mg; sodium 128.9mg.

Refreshing Curd

Prep:

10 mins

Cook:

5 mins

Additional:

2 hrs

Total:

2 hrs 15 mins

Servings:

11

Yield:

1 1/3 cups

Ingredients

1 ½ cups fresh pineapple chunks

2 tablespoons unsalted butter

2 large egg yolks

1 tablespoon cornstarch

2 tablespoons white sugar

1 tablespoon lemon juice

1 pinch salt

Directions

1

Combine pineapple, egg yolks, sugar, lemon juice, cornstarch, and salt in a blender; blend until smooth.

2

Pour into a saucepan and bring to a simmer over medium heat, whisking constantly. Cook and stir until thickened, 3 to 5 minutes.

3

Remove from heat and whisk in butter until fully incorporated. Transfer to a small bowl, cover with plastic wrap, and chill until set, 2 to 3 hours.

Nutrition
Per Serving: 51 calories; protein 0.6g; carbohydrates 6.1g; fat 2.9g; cholesterol 42.8mg; sodium 16.1mg.

Mascarpone Cream

Prep:
15 mins
Total:
15 mins
Servings:
12
Yield:
12 servings

Ingredients

4 each eggs, separated
½ cup white sugar
2 ¼ cups mascarpone cheese
2 tablespoons maple syrup

Directions

1

Whisk egg whites in a stand mixer fitted with a wire whisk attachment until soft peaks form. Set aside in another bowl.

2

Beat egg yolks and sugar together in the bowl using the paddle attachment until smooth and pale. Add maple syrup and beat until fully combined. Slowly mix in mascarpone cheese. Fold in egg whites.

3

Keep in the refrigerator for up to 48 hours, loosely covered with plastic wrap. Cream may begin to separate after 24 hours. Gently stir before serving.

Nutrition

Per Serving: 242 calories; protein 4.8g; carbohydrates 10.7g; fat 21g; cholesterol 107.1mg; sodium 43.3mg.

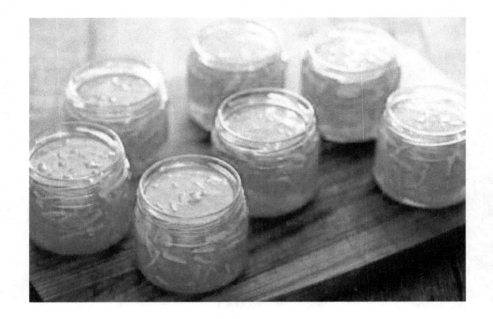

CPSIA information can be obtained
at www.ICGtesting.com
Printed in the USA
BVHW091058260421
605865BV00001B/3